50 things you can do today to manage
stress

Foreword by Jenny Edwards, Vice Chair of the
International Stress Management Association UK

Wendy Green

PERSONAL HEALTH GUIDES

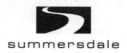
summersdale

50 THINGS YOU CAN DO TODAY TO MANAGE STRESS

Summersdale Publishers Ltd
46 West Street
Chichester
West Sussex
PO19 1RP
UK

www.summersdale.com

Printed and bound in Great Britain

ISBN: 978-1-84953-202-0

Substantial discounts on bulk quantities of Summersdale books are available to corporations, professional associations and other organisations. For details telephone Summersdale Publishers on (+44-1243-771107), fax (+44-1243-786300) or email (nicky@summersdale.com).

Disclaimer
Every effort has been made to ensure that the information in this book is accurate and current at the time of publication. The author and the publisher cannot accept responsibility for any misuse or misunderstanding of any information contained here ACC LIBRARY SERVICES AUSTIN, TX therwise, suffered by any ntained herein. None of the opinions or suggestions in this book is intended to replace medical opinion. If you have concerns about your health, please seek professional advice.

To my husband Gordon,
thanks for being so supportive.

Acknowledgements

I'd like to thank Jennifer Barclay for commissioning this book and for helping me to organise the information. I'd also like to thank Jenny Edwards, Vice Chair of the International Stress Management Association UK, for taking time out of her busy schedule to write the foreword. Thanks also to Emily Kearns and Abbie Headon for their very helpful editorial input.

Other titles in the Personal Health Guides series include:

50 Things You Can Do Today to Increase Your Fertility
50 Things You Can Do Today to Manage Anxiety
50 Things You Can Do Today to Manage Arthritis
50 Things You Can Do Today to Manage Back Pain
50 Things You Can Do Today to Manage Eczema
50 Things You Can Do Today to Manage Fibromyalgia
50 Things You Can Do Today to Manage Hay Fever
50 Things You Can Do Today to Manage IBS
50 Things You Can Do Today to Manage Insomnia
50 Things You Can Do Today to Manage Migraines
50 Things You Can Do Today to Manage Menopause

Contents

1. Learn about stress
2. Keep a stress diary

3. Slow down
4. Say 'no'
5. Cut stress at work
6. De-junk
7. Speed-clean your home
8. Take control of your spending
9. Avoid information overload
10. Follow a simple beauty routine
11. Organise your wardrobe

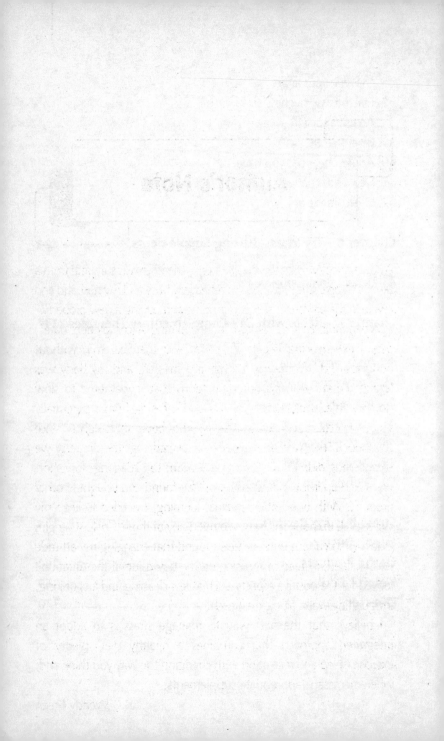

Author's Note

At the time of writing this book a family member was suffering from a serious chronic illness, my job was especially busy and my husband and I were in the process of selling our home and buying a new property.

When problems developed in negotiating a completion date I began experiencing telltale migraines and then eczema; without noticing it I'd become overloaded and stressed, and my body was letting me know in no uncertain terms that it was time to slow down a little. Shortly after that I began suffering from a potentially serious eye condition that was the result of being short-sighted since childhood. Then, to cap it all, we discovered that the property we were buying didn't have vacant possession; to cut a long story short we ended up living in a caravan until we found and bought another property. With two book deadlines looming, I needed to keep my stress levels in check, so I began to put many of the self-help strategies I was writing about into practice. I found that changing my attitude really helped; instead of focusing on the downside of the situation I looked for the positive aspects, such as less cleaning and lots of long, invigorating walks along the beach!

I believe that the best way to manage stress is to adopt an integrated approach that combines a healthy diet, plenty of exercise, sleep and relaxation with changing the way you think and, where necessary, appropriate supplements.

Wendy Green

Foreword

by Jenny Edwards,
Vice Chair of the International Stress Management
Association UK

Stress is a word most of us use in our everyday vocabulary. We read about in newspapers and magazines, hear about it in the news and talk about it amongst our friends, family and work colleagues. However, I usually find that most of us are rather unsure what 'stress' really is, as everyone has their own perception or belief of what it means to them. This excellent book answers that question in an informative and easy-to-read way.

This is a book that provides comprehensive explanations as to the many causes of stress that are particularly relevant to us in today's busy world. What happens to our body when the everyday pressures that we do need to perform and motivate ourselves keep increasing until they are beyond our capacity to cope, is very clearly explained, including the ill health consequence of stress if left unchecked. Perhaps most importantly, this book then provides a guide to help the reader make the necessary changes to redress the balance and shows how we can, with sometimes surprisingly small changes, achieve a better state of well-being.

Today, most of us are time poor, so finding time to read a book can seem like an impossible luxury, especially if we are feeling overwhelmed and stressed; selecting this compact and easy-to-read self-help book could be just the answer. The book is written in a way that allows the reader to dip in and just select a chapter that is of interest, for there is no particular requirement to read it in any order. The comprehensive range of strategies to be found here are provided with detailed explanations and tips that include familiar topics such as diet, exercise and lifestyle, along with chapters on complementary therapies, supplements and some delicious-sounding recipes that I will certainly be trying.

Finding ways to help yourself is very empowering; starting to take some control in your life is a significant step forward towards reducing stress and this excellent book provides at least 50 ways to help you do this. Some of this may seem like common sense, but sometimes we do need to be reminded of the obvious, because the benefits of looking after ourselves today will help to achieve good health in the long term. The mind and body need to work together in order to enjoy all that life has to offer.

Life is a roller coaster… but you do have choices in how you manage it and this well-written self-help book is a really good place to start for yourself and maybe also for a friend.

Introduction

There is plenty of evidence that we are living in stressful times. A report from the Chartered Institute of Personnel and Development in 2011 found that stress is the most common reason for workers taking long-term sickness leave. According to the Health and Safety Executive, stress is the second most commonly reported work-related illness; the mental health charity Mind reports that 500,000 people in the UK believe work-related stress is making them ill and that many of the mental health problems 12 million adults in the UK consult their GP about each year are stress-related. As well as directly affecting our mental and physical health, stress is often responsible for unhealthy habits such as overeating, smoking and drinking too much alcohol, which also take their toll.

This book explains what stress is, the effect it has on the mind and body, and the social, psychological, dietary and lifestyle factors that are thought to contribute to it. It suggests ways that you can reduce the amount of stress in your life to a level that is comfortable for you and how to deal with the stress you can't avoid. It offers a holistic approach and practical advice to help you manage stress.

You will find practical ways to simplify your life to reduce the amount of stress you experience; you'll discover how stress can trigger overindulgence in sugary, salty and fatty foods, which can further stress the body, and how eating a nutritious diet can help you to handle pressure better. You'll learn how being active and sleeping soundly helps the body to combat the effects of stress, as well as the benefits of various types of exercise. Once you have started to feel better through improving your dietary, exercise and sleeping habits, you will find it easier to adopt an anti-stress attitude. Further on in the book there are techniques to help you change the way you view yourself and the situations you encounter, as well as an overview of the supplements that may help you to deal with stress, or help to relieve it. There is also a selection of stress-relieving techniques and treatments from complementary therapies you can try for yourself. At the end of the book you'll find recipes based on the dietary guidelines, as well as details of helpful products, books and organisations.

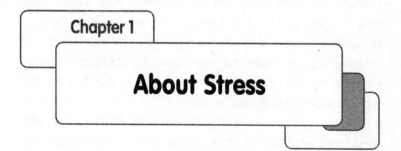

About Stress

This chapter explains what stress is, as well as the differences between pressure and stress. It outlines the three stages of the stress response, and the effects each has on the mind and body. It also considers the causes of modern-day stress including society, biology, work, lifestyle, life changes, psychology and disconnection from nature.

1. Learn about stress

What is stress?

Stress is a term generally used to describe what we feel when we are experiencing too much pressure in our lives. It is usually considered to be a negative and destructive force that can eventually lead to illness.

Pressure usually arises from a positive mental or physical challenge that is within our control and has an end in sight – for example, a work deadline, an exam or a sponsored walk. Often this type of pressure is relatively short-lived and we have an element of control over it; there is usually time for recuperation before the next bout. A little pressure in our lives can be stimulating and challenging; it can motivate us to improve our performance and reach our full potential. Most of us would find life without any kind of pressure boring, and that in itself can be stressful.

According to the HSE (Health and Safety Executive), stress is 'that which arises when the pressure placed upon an individual exceeds the capacity of that individual to cope'.

Excessive pressure usually comes from situations beyond our control that are unrelenting and have no end in sight – such as an unhappy relationship, overwork, chronic illness or unemployment. If you experience this type of pressure over a long period of time, stress hormone levels remain high, causing chemical changes in the body that increase your risk of suffering from physical and psychological symptoms.

What are the effects of stress on the mind and body?

Whilst a little pressure can boost immunity, when we are placed under excessive pressure (stress) hormones like cortisol have a negative effect on immune function, making us more prone to infections, such as colds and flu; allergies, such as hay fever, asthma and eczema; and autoimmune disorders, such as rheumatoid arthritis. Long-term stress can also cause irritability, depression and anxiety, which can lead to relationship problems and further stress.

We all have our own individual levels and types of pressure we feel comfortable with – what is challenging and motivating for one person might be completely overwhelming for another. Also, we all react to stress in different ways – some people suffer from emotional or behavioural symptoms, while others develop physical problems, or a mixture of both. It is important to understand both the difference between pressure and stress, and how much pressure you are able to handle at any one time. It is also vital that you learn to recognise your individual early signs and symptoms so that you can take steps to reduce your stress levels before they cause you serious harm.

What is the stress response?

The stress response is basically how the body responds when confronted with what the brain perceives to be a stressful situation. The stress response has three stages:

1. **Alarm** – this involves the 'fight or flight' response.

2. **Adaptation** – if the stressful situation isn't resolved, your body uses all of its resources to adapt, and you are likely to suffer from physical and mental symptoms.

3. **Exhaustion** – this is where the body has used up its resources and you are at risk of suffering from more serious health conditions.

Alarm stage

When faced with what you perceive as a stressful situation the sympathetic nervous system takes over to trigger the alarm stage of the stress response. This is designed to enable us to deal with difficult, or even dangerous, situations and involves the brain preparing the body to either stay put to face the perceived threat, or to escape from it. This worked well in primitive times when you might have to deal with a passing threat or danger fairly quickly, but unfortunately the situations that induce the stress response (stressors) nowadays are unlikely to require either of these responses, and can happen more often and continue for longer. The 'fight or flight' response triggered at the alarm stage invokes these reactions in the body:

Adrenal glands release stress hormones cortisol, noradrenaline and adrenaline.

Heart rate speeds up.

 Liver releases energy stored as glycogen.

 Blood sugar rises.

 Cholesterol level rises.

 Blood pressure rises.

 Breathing becomes faster and shallower.

 Sweating increases.

 Blood vessels close.

 Digestion slows down or speeds up.

More white blood cells are released, increasing immune function.

Fibrin, a substance that promotes blood clotting is released into the bloodstream.

You may notice these physical signs of acute stress:

 Forehead tenses.

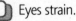 Eyes strain.

 Jaws and teeth clench.

Skin tightens.

 Mouth dries up.

Anger/hostility.

Butterflies in stomach.

Adaptation

Your body is under strain as it harnesses its resources to adapt to chronic stress. During this stage the body continues to produce stress hormones to provide energy to deal with the situation. Stress hormones affect the way the immune system functions – increasing the risk of infections, autoimmune and allergic conditions. Over time the effects of this stage of the stress response include:

Physical

 Sleep problems

 Tiredness

Muscular aches and pains, especially in the neck, shoulders and back

Headaches/migraines

 Irritable bowel syndrome (IBS)

 Indigestion

Skin conditions, e.g. eczema, psoriasis

 Asthma

 Allergies

 Food intolerances

 Weight gain/weight loss

 Panic attacks/nausea

 Minor infections, e.g. colds/sore throats, due to reduced immunity

 Palpitations

 Menstrual changes

 Loss of libido

Mental

 Difficulty making decisions

 Poor performance

Lack of concentration

Forgetfulness

Panic attacks

Emotional

 Blaming yourself

 Feeling inadequate

 Dwelling on the past

 Worry

 Inability to relax

 Feeling tense and anxious

 Impatience

 Irritability

 Losing your temper easily

 Tearfulness

 Poor sense of humour

Behavioural

 Recklessness

 Smoking more

 Drinking more alcohol

Using recreational drugs

Poor appetite/overeating

Craving sugary, fatty or salty foods

Talking too quickly

Outbursts of anger

Avoiding contact with other people

Nervous habits, e.g. nail biting, hair pulling, fist clenching, foot tapping, blinking and nervous tics

Exhaustion

The body has used up its physical and emotional resources. The constant bombardment from stress hormones over a long period of time has reduced levels of important brain chemicals, impaired immune function, raised blood pressure and cholesterol levels, and increased blood clotting, leaving the body at risk of more serious health problems. These can include the following:

 Depression

High blood pressure

Irregular heartbeat (arrhythmia)

Obesity

Coronary heart disease

Stroke

Diabetes

Cancer

Rheumatoid arthritis

Menstrual problems, such as premenstrual syndrome (PMS)

Fertility problems

Thyroid disorders

Stomach ulcers

How does stress affect the immune system?

In short bursts, stress can stimulate the immune response. However, chronic stress can compromise the immune response, leaving you more prone to infections and viruses; yet paradoxically it can also trigger excessive immune activity, leading to allergies like eczema and autoimmune conditions, such as rheumatoid arthritis and lupus.

Researchers believe this is because stress hormones such as cortisol affect the balance of cytokines, which are a type of white blood cell involved in the immune response. After a while Th1 cytokines are reduced, leaving the body more prone to infections, while Th2 cytokine levels are raised; higher levels of Th2 cytokines are linked to inflammation, and increased allergic and autoimmune responses. This helps to explain why, after a period of stress, people often catch a cold or flu, or those with allergies or autoimmune diseases tend to experience flare-ups.

Another factor is that stressed people often turn to junk food, caffeine, alcohol and nicotine to help them cope, and often suffer from sleep problems – all of which can compromise immune function.

Clearly stress can have a serious negative impact on your physical and mental health, therefore managing it should be considered an integral part of a healthy lifestyle.

What causes stress?

Human beings have always experienced stress, but nowadays the types of stresses and strains we encounter in everyday life are different to those our ancestors might have had to deal with; thousands of years ago stressors commonly faced were probably a lack of food or shelter, or even a close encounter with a wild animal. Today most of us in the Western world have plenty to eat and drink, and a roof over our heads, but fast-paced modern-day living poses a host of completely different problems, ranging from being stuck in a traffic jam, to divorce, losing your job and worries about debt.

Society

Society is more aspirational and materialistic than ever before and, as a result, we are constantly striving to look, feel and do better, and are working longer and harder to earn more money. Consequently, many of us are overloaded and experiencing stress.

The combination of juggling a job with childcare and possibly caring for elderly parents, as well as shouldering most of the domestic chores, leaves many women stressed; men, too, often have to juggle work with helping to care for young children. The current economic downturn means many are struggling with losing their jobs and finding themselves unable to provide for their families. Young people also face increasing pressures not only in terms of educational achievement, but also from bullying, parental divorce, drug and alcohol abuse, and difficulties finding a job.

Our relationships with our partner, family members and friends can be sources of stress, especially when facing relationship breakdown or divorce, bereavement, and problems with childcare etc. On the other hand, being happily married and/or having a good social network can help you to cope with stress better.

Biology

A poll of 2,000 people carried out by the Stroke Association and Siemens in 2011 found that nearly twice as many women as men felt their stress levels were out of control.

This is possibly because women's biology predisposes them to take on a nurturing role and to multitask, both of which can lead to stress. According to leading American gynaecologists Dr Stephanie McClellan and Dr Beth Hamilton, who have spent years studying the way women's nervous systems react to stress hormones, women also release more stress hormones than men and they stay in their bodies for longer.

Work

A report by the Institute of Personnel & Development in 2011 cited job insecurity caused by the economic downturn, an excessive workload, poor management and restructuring in the workplace as the leading causes of work-related stress.

Work can be stressful, especially if you have little control over your work situation, work long hours or shifts, don't have time to take breaks, have a heavy workload, or too much responsibility. Lack of help and support from your co-workers or supervisors and worries about job security can all take their toll. Other causes of work-related stress include lack of opportunities to advance, and doing a job that is boring and repetitive.

Many people are working longer and longer hours, often without breaks, in the hope of impressing their managers and holding on to their jobs. Unfortunately, working in this way is likely to increase your stress levels, which could hamper your performance and make you more susceptible to illness, therefore reducing your productivity.

Lifestyle

Poor eating habits, lack of exercise, and insufficient relaxation and good-quality sleep can stress the body and affect the way it deals with stress. Overindulgence in caffeine and alcohol can also increase stress levels, and affect the way we cope with everyday pressures.

Life changes

Life changes are a source of stress because change involves dealing with the unknown, which most people find stressful, and often they are caused by events out of our control such as bereavement or redundancy. Listed on the next page are the life events most likely to cause stress.

Psychology

Psychologists believe that most stress is the result of our self-image and individual perception of events, rather than the events themselves. For example, a person with a positive self-image and outlook is less likely to feel threatened by difficult situations and powerless to address problems than someone with lower self-esteem. A negative outlook can contribute to stress. Your personality type can also determine how much stress you experience; people with 'Type A' personalities tend to be perfectionists who are very driven, rushed, ambitious and time-conscious – traits which can increase the risk of experiencing stress. 'Type B' personalities are more relaxed, less driven and time-conscious and much less prone to stress.

Holmes & Rahe Stress Scale (1967)

Highest stress rating	High stress rating	Moderate stress rating	Lower stress rating
Death of partner	Reconciliation	Family arguments	Change in working conditions
Divorce or separation	Retirement	Taking on a large mortgage	Change of schools
Prison sentence	Serious ill health in the family	Legal action over debt	Holidays
Death of a close relative	Pregnancy	New responsibilities at work	Change in contact with relatives
Personal injury or illness	Sexual problems	Child starting/ finishing school	Minor violations of the law
Marriage	New baby/ family member	Son/daughter leaving home	Joining/ leaving a social group
Loss of job	Change of job	Difficulties with in-laws	Christmas
Moving house	Money problems	Change in living conditions	Small mortgage/ loan
	Death of a close friend	Problems with boss	

Disconnection from nature

Recent studies suggest that city dwellers experience more stress than those living in rural settings. Pollution, noise, crowding, heavy traffic and the faster pace of living in urban areas could all contribute. Some researchers argue that man has a natural affinity with nature and modern society's 'disconnection' from the natural world is a major cause of stress.

Does stress affect men and women differently?

While both men and women experience the alarm, adaptation and exhaustion stages of the stress response, women's biology slightly modifies this process. This both predisposes women to experience more stress and affects the way they deal with it.

Women are more likely to become stressed than men because their brains are programmed to multitask, and take responsibility for the care and well-being of others. Studies suggest women release more stress hormones when under pressure and these stay in their bodies for longer than they do in men's. Research suggests that women not only release cortisol and adrenaline when under stress, but also oxytocin, a chemical that makes them want to 'tend and befriend'. The researchers put this 'tend and befriend' reaction to stress down to Stone Age women needing to protect their children from predators and to join forces with other women in order to survive.

The need to nurture (tend) when under pressure means women often take on too much, which makes them even more stressed. However, the befriending instinct makes women want to talk to others when they are feeling stressed, which lowers cortisol levels, making them feel calmer. This helps to explain why social support appears to help women to deal with stress more than it does men and why women tend to want to talk things over when they are stressed, while men are more likely to retreat.

Before the menopause, women are less likely to suffer from stress-related heart disease than men, probably because of the protective effects of oestrogen. The risk of heart disease increases after the menopause when oestrogen levels fall dramatically.

Men's reaction to stress tends to be mainly the fight or flight one – either react aggressively or escape from the situation. This is why they are less likely to open up to others when they are feeling tense and are more likely to try to escape from a stressful situation to help them cope. They might do this by engaging in a sport such as golf or fishing, or in risky behaviour; research at the University of Southern California in 2009 suggested that men often deal with stress by drinking heavily, driving too fast, smoking, gambling, taking drugs or having extra-marital affairs.

Research suggests that the impact of stress on men and women's immune systems is also different. A recent study of 1,200 office workers found that when men were stressed at work they were more likely to develop a cold than women were. This might be because women have stronger immune systems with more white 'fighter' cells. Women's more robust immune systems might be one of the reasons why they are more likely to develop autoimmune disorders such as lupus and rheumatoid arthritis as a result of stress.

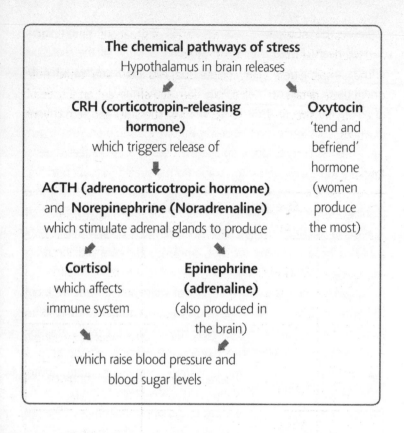

The chemical pathways of stress
Hypothalamus in brain releases

CRH (corticotropin-releasing hormone)
which triggers release of

ACTH (adrenocorticotropic hormone)
and **Norepinephrine (Noradrenaline)**
which stimulate adrenal glands to produce

Cortisol
which affects
immune system

Epinephrine (adrenaline)
(also produced in
the brain)

which raise blood pressure and
blood sugar levels

Oxytocin
'tend and
befriend'
hormone
(women
produce
the most)

2. Keep a stress diary

The best place to start when looking to reduce the amount of stress and overload in your life is to identify your stressors. Sometimes when we're feeling under pressure we lose sight of what's really going on in our lives. Taking stock and identifying the areas of your life that could be contributing to your stress levels will enable you to do something about it.

For a couple of weeks, record the details of situations, times, places and people that make you feel stressed.

The sample Stress Diary below suggests how you could note down these details, as well as rate each stressful event on a scale of one (slightly stressful) to ten (extremely stressful) and record your reactions.

Date:

Time	Stressful event	Stress rating (1-10)	Reaction
8.30am	Stuck in traffic jam	8	Panicked about being late for work. Tense neck & shoulder muscles.
9.30 am	Arrived at work 30 minutes late	8	Arrived at meeting late. Aching neck and shoulder muscles.
12 noon	Missed lunch break to catch up on tasks	9	Throbbing headache.

After a couple of weeks, read through your diary to see if there are certain stressful situations you experience more than others. Once you've identified these, think about each one and ask yourself: 'Can I avoid it?' To take the traffic jam example, perhaps you could avoid rush-hour traffic by using an alternative route, or making the journey earlier or later? To take another small example, if you find doing the weekly shop at the supermarket stressful, perhaps you could avoid it by doing your shopping online?

If you cannot avoid a particular stressor, you can usually reduce the level of stress you experience by taking practical steps to help you cope better, such as eating well, taking exercise and getting plenty of sleep, or by changing your attitude towards the situation. You can reduce your overall stress levels by simplifying your life. You can also relieve the effects of stress by taking time out for yourself, practising relaxation techniques and doing things that help you unwind. This book aims to offer you practical advice in all of these areas to help you both reduce and relieve stress.

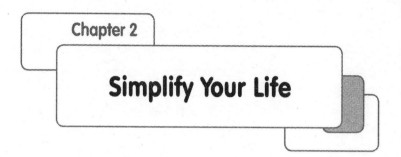

Chapter 2

Simplify Your Life

The life we live today is far more complex than that of our parents and grandparents. We have much more choice than ever before in almost every area of our lives – from TV and radio channels to consumer products like foods, cosmetics, cleaning products, holidays and technology. Although it may essentially be a good thing, being faced with a bewildering array of products and services to choose from can be stressful and time consuming. Where in the past there were one or two brands of a product there are now often dozens. Everything we buy involves a decision – regular, low-salt, low-fat or low-sugar? Perfumed, unperfumed or hypoallergenic? Caffeinated or decaffeinated? Organic or non-organic? Fresh, frozen or tinned?

Modern society is also far more aspirational and materialistic than it was fifty years ago. We're constantly bombarded by the media and advertisers with images of the so-called perfect life – slim, beautiful people in designer clothes, driving top-of-the-range cars and living in big houses, full of material goods like widescreen TVs and the latest computer. For most of us this kind of lifestyle isn't attainable, but it leaves us feeling we must always strive for more.

This 'have-it-all' attitude necessitates living our lives at an ever faster pace, as we work longer and longer hours to achieve a better lifestyle. Today's society expects women to juggle full- or part-time work with motherhood, a happy relationship and running a home, while possibly caring for an ailing parent, and ensuring they always look attractive. As a result, many of us are 'cash rich' but' time poor', fitting in gym sessions and hairdresser appointments in our lunch hours – that's if we can find the time to take them. Evenings and weekends are spent desperately trying to catch up with household chores, and spending time with family and friends.

Higher divorce rates and fewer people choosing to marry means there are four times more people living alone than during the 1950s. Single, divorced or separated people – especially lone parents – are more likely to suffer from financial worries as they struggle to survive on a single wage and bring up children alone. In short, our lives have become so overloaded we are paying the price, with more and more of us succumbing to stress and stress-related illnesses.

This chapter suggests practical ways you can simplify your life to reduce stress levels, including slowing down, delegating, cutting work-related stress, de-cluttering, speed-cleaning, taking control of your spending, avoiding information overload, adopting a simple beauty routine and organising your wardrobe.

3. Slow down

Many of us are living our lives at a faster and faster pace as we juggle a career, relationships, family and domestic commitments with a hectic social life. This constant sense of urgency makes us impatient and frustrated when we have to stop and wait, maybe in a queue or a traffic jam, or when the bus or train is late, raising our stress levels unnecessarily.

Try this:
Next time you're caught up in a queue or a traffic jam, or your bus or train is delayed, try looking upon the time you spend waiting as a welcome break from rushing around. Do something relaxing like deep breathing, listening to your favourite radio station or reading.

Accept you'll never get everything done
If you constantly push yourself to complete everything on your to-do list, thinking you'll be able to relax when you cross off the last task, remember you'll never get everything done; as soon as you complete tasks more will replace them.

Try this:
Ask: 'What are the three most important tasks I need to complete today?' Then make sure you complete them first.

Ask for help

Don't think you always have to do everything yourself. When you feel overloaded with tasks, ask for help. Ask your partner and children to help with household chores, and don't be too proud to accept offers of help from colleagues at work.

4. Say 'no'
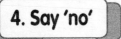

If it feels like your life is spiralling out of control through too many demands from work, home, your partner, family and friends, perhaps it is time to streamline your life. If you regularly feel under pressure and stressed due to a lack of time, try reviewing how you use it.

Keep a diary for a few days to see how you spend your time, then decide which activities you can do less often, or even stop doing altogether, to make more time for the things that are most important to you. Say 'no' to non-essential tasks you don't have time for, or just don't want to do. It's a little word, but it can cut your stress levels dramatically. If you find it hard to say 'no', consider brushing up on your assertiveness skills (see Chapter 5).

5. Cut stress at work

The following steps, aimed at making your working day less pressurised, could help you avoid, or at least reduce, the amount of stress you experience at work.

Prepare for work

Prepare for work the night before by getting your clothes and any work equipment ready. If you can never decide what to wear, try having a specific outfit for each day of the week, so that you don't have to worry about it. Plan what you will eat for breakfast and prepare your packed lunch to save time in the morning.

Adjust your workspace

To avoid tension in the neck and shoulders, perfect your posture by adjusting your work area. If you work with a computer screen it should be straight ahead, so you don't have to twist your neck or shoulders. You should be able to see the screen sitting upright, not leaning forward or back. The top of the screen should be in line with your eyes. Your upper arms should be at your sides and your wrists and forearms should be horizontal when you use your keyboard. Adjust your seat height if you need to. Your pelvis should be a little higher than your knees. Your feet should be flat on the floor – if you can't manage this, use a shallow footrest. If you're not sure whether your workspace is suited to your needs, ask your employers to check it for you, to ensure that it complies with health and safety regulations.

Avoid second-hand stress at work

Professor Elaine Hatfield, a psychologist from the University of Hawaii, claimed recently that stress in the workplace can be contagious – if a colleague is stressed you can unconsciously 'absorb' their negative emotions. To avoid 'catching' stress when a colleague is complaining about their work or personal life try to say something positive about their situation, or offer to help them. If they persist in being negative try taking a break – perhaps by going to make a cup of tea. If you can't walk away, make a conscious effort to stay positive and avoid adopting your colleague's mindset.

Buy a plant

Surprisingly, recent research at Washington State University reported that having a plant on your desk at work can cut stress levels, lower blood pressure and boost productivity. These benefits are thought to be down to the calming effects of nature, as well as the air-purifying and humidifying effects of plants. Foliage plants are thought to work better than flowering plants because they produce the most oxygen.

Manage your workload

If you're feeling stressed out because you have a lot of work to get through, try these techniques to help you manage your workload and stay in control.

De-clutter your desk

De-cluttering your desk makes it easier to concentrate on your task in hand. Sort through any paperwork and decide what to do with it; if it needs to be acted on put it in your in-tray to be dealt with as soon as possible; if you will need it at a later date, file it away where you can find it easily; if it is out of date, or no longer needed, bin it.

Write a to-do list

Write a to-do list at the end of each working day, ready for the next day. When you have a long to-do list, number tasks in terms of urgency and importance, then carry them out in that order. Cross off tasks as soon as you complete them.

Chunk

If you have a few telephone calls to make, letters to write or emails to respond to, try 'chunking'. Chunking is where you set aside a period of time to complete similar tasks together.

De-stress at work

Socialise

While too many interruptions from emails, phone calls, text messages and colleagues chatting can lead to work piling up, being sociable at work has been shown to reduce stress. So take five minutes for a cuppa and a chat, if you can, during your working day.

Take a break

No matter how busy you are you should make time for one or two short breaks during your working day. Going for a walk or even just reading a newspaper – preferably away from your desk – can take your mind off work and lower your stress levels.

Stretch

Stretching your body every hour or two helps to prevent muscular tension from developing and gets the blood flowing, helping to prevent blood clots. Even just walking to the kitchen or going to the photocopier can help. If you don't have time to leave your desk, try these 'desk stretches' from your chair.

- Clench your calf and thigh muscles, hold, then release. Repeat two or three times.

- Stretch your legs out in front of you, toes pointing upwards, hold for one minute. Repeat.

- Sit with your feet directly in line with your knees. Raise both feet and hold for one minute. Repeat.

- Slowly tilt your head towards your left shoulder. Next tilt your head towards the right. Repeat on each side several times.

Lift and tense both shoulders and hold for ten seconds. Allow them to fall and relax. Repeat three times.

 Circle each shoulder alternately two or three times – first forwards and then backwards.

 Place the backs of your hands on your lower back. Arch your back by pushing your hips forward and pulling your shoulders back. Hold for ten seconds and repeat up to three times.

 Stretch both arms out in front of you at shoulder height, palms upright. Bend forearms back and touch your shoulders with your fingertips. Repeat up to five times.

 Clench your fists tightly for five seconds. Stretch your fingers out, then relax them. Repeat up to five times.

Switch off!

Switch off from work after hours by turning off your mobile phone and Blackberry, and avoiding checking your emails. If you have to bring your work things home with you, put them away so that they remain out of sight and out of mind.

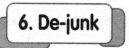

6. De-junk

A crammed wardrobe, heaving shelves and overflowing cupboards can raise stress levels as you struggle to find things. De-junking your home can save you time and energy, and leave you feeling calmer and more in control.

If you haven't worn, read, or used an item for two years or more, donate it to a charity shop, recycle it through Freegle, Freecycle or Clothes for Cash (see Directory), sell it on eBay, or bin it. If you have a lot of items to sort through enlist the help of your partner, a family member or a friend, if you can, or try tackling one room at a time. Don't forget to de-clutter the bathroom – throw away any pots or tubes you haven't used for months.

De-cluttering can be hard work, but the results are worthwhile; not only will you have a sense of achievement, but you may also have helped a worthwhile cause or boosted your bank balance. But, most importantly, you'll be amazed at how much more at ease you feel when your house is clutter-free.

Try this:
If you can't bear to part with an item, store it under a bed or in the loft. Make a rule that if you haven't wanted to use it or wear it within a year, you will get rid of it.

Tips for a tidy home
Once you've cleared the clutter, try these tips to stop it building up again:

1. Keep a waste bin in each room.

2. Ensure you have plenty of cupboards, boxes and shelves for storage.

3. Ask everyone in the house to tidy up after themselves.

4. Bin newspapers and letters you don't need to keep as soon as you have read them.

7. Speed-clean your home

Juggling household chores with a job and caring for a family can be a major source of stress.

For stress-free cleaning tackle just a couple of rooms at a time, rather than the whole house.

 Clean first, then vacuum.

 Clean the dirtiest room first.

 Wear an apron with pockets, so that you can carry your cleaners, cloths and dusters around with you.

 Clean from left to right, top to bottom and from the back of an object to the front – with no doubling back.

Only clean areas that look dirty, i.e. don't clean a whole door – just wipe where you can see marks.

If you only have ten minutes before a visitor is due to arrive...

◯ Whisk a feather duster or an absorbent cloth over the furniture, mantelpiece and windowsill.

◯ Quickly sweep or vacuum the floor.

◯ Fluff up the pile on any rugs with your hand.

◯ Plump up and straighten any cushions.

◯ Light one or two scented candles.

8. Take control of your spending

'Annual income twenty pounds, annual expenditure nineteen six, result happiness. Annual income twenty pounds, annual expenditure twenty pounds ought and six, result misery.'

Charles Dickens, *David Copperfield*

Overspending and debt can be a major source of stress – especially in today's materialistic times. An online survey of more than 1,400 people in the UK by the Really Worried website in 2008 found that the top concern was the cost of living, closely followed by energy prices, debt and pensions. Cutting down on spending reduces the risk of becoming debt-ridden and falling prey to the stress that money problems can cause.

Aspiring to a lifestyle we can't really afford and buying items we don't really need simply because 'we deserve it' can lead to spiralling personal debts; credit cards have made it far too easy for us to spend far more than we can afford. If your prime focus in life is the pursuit of material goods you could end up working longer and longer hours to earn the money to pay for them, and becoming more and more stressed in the process.

Reassessing how you spend your money and taking control of your finances could help you avoid the burden of money worries and enable you to live the life you want, whether that is changing jobs, cutting your working hours, or even retiring.

1. **Set yourself a realistic budget**

   Set yourself a realistic budget and stick to it. Work out how much money you need to cover your essential outgoings, such as food, mortgage/rent, heating, electricity, insurance and travel. Check to see if you can save money by switching your mortgage lender or energy supplier. Pay off any debts. If you are struggling to meet credit card or mortgage payments always speak to your lender and try to negotiate an amount you can manage to pay.

2. **Spend your money on what matters most to you**

   Avoid falling into the trap of spending money on things you don't really want, simply because of social expectations or to cheer yourself up; far from being a source of comfort, overindulging in 'retail therapy' can be a major cause of stress when you are faced with a huge credit card bill. Decide what matters most to you and then spend your money accordingly. For example, if you love having a nice home perhaps you could direct more of your resources towards that by cutting out another major expense, such as running a car; if your local public transport services are adequate and you don't have to commute far to work, do you really need one?

3. **Try to live more frugally**

   Do you need a wardrobe crammed with clothes, half of which you will never wear? Do you need to use the most expensive brands of cosmetics and perfumes? If you enjoy eating out could you reduce it to a weekly treat and perhaps make the most of local 'early-bird' deals? Could you swap books with friends when you have read them, or make use of your local library? If you enjoy holidays, check online for the cheapest deals. Focus on rewarding activities that don't cost a lot – anything from walking, to going to free concerts, or visiting free art galleries and museums – so long as you enjoy it and it helps you focus on 'being' rather than 'having.' Living in this way will enable you to spend less, but still afford the things you enjoy.

4. **Work out how much you can afford to spend on food**

   Food is increasingly expensive, but is the cornerstone of good health. Work out how much you can afford to spend on nourishing yourself and your family, and then aim to buy food for a balanced diet (see Chapter 3). Identify what you need and make a list before you shop.

   If you're on a tight budget, focus on meals containing cheap but nutritious ingredients, such as fruit and vegetables, pulses, potatoes, brown rice, wholemeal bread, pasta and oats. Eggs, baked beans, tinned sardines and tuna are all good-value sources of protein and other nutrients. These foods can form the basis of family meals – such as stir-fries, broths, casseroles and pasta dishes. You can save money on these basic foods at the cheaper supermarkets or by buying in bulk – take advantage of 'two-for-one' or other special offers. Compare food prices at different supermarkets. Look out for foods that are priced down because they are close to the sell-by date. Your local market can often be cheaper – especially at the end of the day, or on a Saturday.

Make your own cheaper and healthier versions of ready meals by cooking extra portions of your favourite dishes and freezing them.

Growing your own vegetables can save a lot of money and you will reap the health benefits of eating produce that is not only pesticide-free, but also fresher than that bought in the supermarket. You don't need a big garden or an allotment – you can grow various vegetables including potatoes, carrots, peas, tomatoes, beetroot and broad, French and runner beans in pots or containers. Use a deep pot or container and add stones or broken pots to aid drainage; then fill with compost, before planting and watering.

Taking a home-made sandwich or salad, plus fruit and yogurt, to work, is far healthier and cheaper than buying lunch. If you forgo that daily takeaway cappuccino, too, you could save quite a bit each month.

Ask: 'Do I need this, or do I just want it?' before you buy. You'll probably find you've been spending more money than you need to.

Try this:
When you go shopping make it a rule not to buy on impulse. If you see something you like, go home and think about it. If you decide it's something you really need you can go back later to buy it.

9. Avoid information overload

We are constantly bombarded with information through TV, radio, print media, texts, emails and the Internet. This means the brain is continuously stimulated with images, facts and ideas that it has to process. Psychologists have termed this 'infomania'. Research from the University of London concluded that the effects of constant texting and emailing throughout the day on the brain's functioning are similar to those caused by losing a night's sleep; if your brain is constantly 'on standby' for the next message or piece of information it can affect your productivity as it can only deal with one thing at a time – and it can even lower your IQ.

Television

TV can be addictive: the more programmes you watch, the more you want to watch, and there are more TV stations and programmes on offer than ever before. News is broadcast 24/7, so it is tempting to have the TV on all the time. While watching TV can be relaxing, entertaining and informative, too much can crowd out other enjoyable and enriching activities, including talking to your partner and children. Not only that, TV tends to promote the materialism and perfectionism that leads to stress and overload.

Solution: Be selective about your TV viewing – choose the programmes you really want to watch and either watch them live or record them to view later. Switch the TV off when there is nothing that really interests you and do something else with your precious time.

Email

Reading and responding to emails can take up a lot of time; no sooner have we read all of the emails in our inbox than another dozen or so appear. A lot of personal emails are unsolicited junk mail or email offers from online companies we have previously bought items from, and sometimes it is hard to resist opening them just in case they are offering us the deal of a lifetime.

Solution: Make it a rule that you only check your personal emails a couple of times a day. Ensure the spam filter is always on and, if any junk emails slip through, discipline yourself to delete them without opening them. As soon as you have answered an email either file it away in a folder or delete it.

Internet

The Internet is a great source of information and entertainment, but if you find yourself surfing for hours on end, you could be frittering away time you could be spending following other interests. It is also so easy to get hooked on Internet shopping, and before you know it you have a hefty credit card bill for stuff you don't need and little time for real life! Twitter, Facebook and other social-networking sites are free and can be useful, so long as you don't spend hours and hours of your spare time using them rather than meeting members of your family and friends face to face.

Solution: Set yourself a time limit for online browsing each day and aim to stick to it. Use the time you save to do the things you keep saying you don't have time for.

10. Follow a simple beauty routine

Looking your best can increase your confidence and cut your stress levels, so long as you keep your beauty routine simple.

There are more beauty products to choose from than ever before, but all your skin and hair really need is to be cleansed and moisturised.

Speedy skin care

Rather than following a complicated skin care routine that involves lots of different products and time, focus on the four key steps – cleansing, exfoliating, toning and moisturising, and use just one skin care product that can multitask.

Step 1: Massage in lotion or cream to cleanse.

Step 2: Remove with a damp flannel or muslin cloth to exfoliate.

Step 3: Splash with cold water to tone.

Step 4: Reapply cream or lotion to moisturise.

A light lotion like Nivea or, if your skin is dry, Pond's Cold Cream, can be used as a facial cleanser, eye make-up remover, moisturiser, body lotion, hand cream and even as a hydrating face mask if you apply extra: leave it on while you're in the bath or shower and then rinse it off with tepid water.

Easy hair care

Select a style that suits your type of hair and emphasises natural curls, waves or straight hair, so that you don't spend hours battling against nature with straighteners, perms, or lots of styling products.

Wash your hair every other day, rather than every day – not only will you save time, but your hair will also be in better condition because of less exposure to heat from the hairdryer, as well as shampoo and other hair products – all of which strip away natural oils. If your hair becomes oily in between washes, massage in a little talc or spray with a dry shampoo, such as Batiste, then brush out.

Despite what it says on the bottle, shampooing once is usually enough.

If you're in a rush and don't have much time to wash your hair, clip or tie your hair back then just wash the fringe and parting areas, where the grease is most noticeable. This is especially time-saving if you have medium to long hair, as it dramatically cuts down on the time spent drying your hair, yet leaves it looking freshly washed.

'No tears' baby shampoo has a multitude of uses: you can use it not only to wash your hair but also as a body wash, foam bath, face wash and eye make-up remover, and lathered up when you shave your legs.

If you're in a rush, use leave-in conditioner to avoid having to rinse your hair twice.

Use fewer cosmetics
Using lots of different cosmetics can take up too much of your precious time, especially when you need to be out of the door in a hurry. Keeping the number of products you use to a minimum will help you achieve speedy glamour, and will also be better for both your skin and your pocket.

Dot and blend in foundation only where your skin needs cover – or, if your skin is oily, dust mineral powder over shiny areas and repeat during the day if needed.

Choose a bronze-coloured cream blusher that will multitask as an eye shadow and a lip tint.

Have your eyelashes and eyebrows professionally tinted, so you don't need to apply mascara and eyebrow pencil every day.

Natural nails

Nail varnish tends to chip fairly quickly, so it needs to be removed and reapplied often, which is time consuming. Buffing your nails to a shine offers a time-saving and more natural alternative – you can carry a nail buffer around with you and use it whenever you have a spare moment.

Time-saving grooming tips for men

- Opt for an all-in-one hair and body wash rather than individual products for your body, face and hair.

- Shave in the shower using a multiblade (non-electric) razor. The steam from the shower softens the beard and helps the razor glide over the skin.

- Use a multitasking nappy-rash cream like Sudocrem to soothe razor burn and treat acne, eczema and sweat rash.

11. Organise your wardrobe

Deciding what to wear can be time-consuming, especially if your wardrobe is disorganised and you can't ever find what you are looking for.

If you often think 'what on earth shall I wear for work tomorrow?', opt for a basic work wardrobe of smart black or grey skirt or trouser suits, or pinafore or tailored shift dresses. Ring the changes by teaming them with different coloured blouses or shirts.

Hang your clothes in sections in your wardrobe according to what you wear them for – for example, hang all the clothes you wear for work together, then do the same for your casual wear and your 'going out' clothes. Within each section group clothes of the same colour together. This enables you to find the type of outfit you want in the colour/s you want much more quickly and easily.

Cut down on the time you spend ironing by buying clothes made from 'no iron' or 'easy iron' fabrics.

Store your shoes in pairs on a shoe rack at the bottom of the wardrobe so that you spot the ones you want easily.

Take some 'me time'

Set aside some of the time you've saved for yourself. Use it to do something you enjoy – it could be anything from luxuriating in a warm, scented bath, to reading a book by your favourite author, or going for a walk – anything that helps you to switch off from your responsibilities and unwind.

Chapter 3

Eat a De-Stress Diet

Stress can lead to poor eating habits, which can cause nutritional deficiencies that stress your body further. This will hamper your body's ability to deal with stress, so it is important to ensure you eat a balanced diet.

When you are stressed you are more likely to crave high-energy, sugary and fatty foods, such as sweets and pastries. During the stress response, cortisol is produced to trigger the release of extra energy in the blood in the form of sugars and fats, to enable the body to fight or take flight. However, it also blocks the release of leptin, a hormone that tells us when we are full, and insulin, so that we feel hungrier than usual and eat more. If you don't do something to burn off the extra calories you are likely to gain weight – especially around the middle, because if the extra energy isn't used up the body stores it as fat around the middle, close to the liver, so it can be quickly converted back into energy if it is needed. Unfortunately, most stressful situations in the twenty-first century don't necessitate fighting or running away, hence stress can lead to weight gain.

Another problem with sugary foods is that they provide quick bursts of energy, which are followed by fatigue, as blood sugar levels fall, making us crave more sugar. Prolonged stress can also lead to the adrenal glands producing insufficient stress hormones, which can disrupt salt levels and trigger cravings for salty foods such as crisps, salted peanuts etc. Stress causes the body to use up more nutrients than usual, so a poor diet may cause deficiencies, leading to further stress and health problems. Also, when you're stressed and lack the time or energy to cook nourishing meals you're more likely to grab fast food or a ready meal – the types of food that are often high in fat, salt and sugar, and low in nutrients. Or you might be so busy that you miss meals to save time, but end up feeling so hungry that you grab whatever is at hand.

This chapter looks at how eating a balanced, low-glycaemic index (GI) diet can keep your blood sugar stable, and your emotions on an even keel, to help you deal with stressful situations better. Protein foods and their role in the production of neurotransmitters (the brain's 'chemical messengers') are discussed. It also outlines the healthy fats, vitamins and minerals that you need to give you energy as well as support your nervous and immune systems when you are stressed. During periods of stress many of us turn to caffeine to give us a boost, or alcohol to calm us down; we'll see the effects this has on our mind and body. You will find recipes based on many of the eating guidelines in this chapter at the end of the book.

12. Go for low-GI foods

Your brain needs a steady supply of glucose (sugar) to enable it to work efficiently and deal with everyday life. Fluctuations in blood sugar levels can affect the brain, causing mood swings and anxiety. Also, low blood sugar levels trigger the stress response, as the body reacts by producing adrenaline to stimulate the release of glucose into the bloodstream.

The glycaemic index (GI) is a measure of how quickly a food raises the level of sugar in the blood. Choosing foods with a low glycaemic index is thought to be the best way to maintain steady glucose levels and keep your emotions on an even keel.

Carbohydrates with a high GI are easily broken down into glucose, causing your blood sugar to rise quickly and then fall just as fast. Refined, processed foods such as white bread, cakes, biscuits, pastries, sugary drinks and sweets usually have a high GI. Carbohydrates with a low GI take longer to digest, allowing your blood glucose to rise slowly and steadily. Unrefined, complex carbohydrates, such as wholegrain bread, porridge, wholewheat pasta, brown basmati rice, barley, sweet potatoes, sweetcorn, carrots, beans, lentils, peas, apples, pears and oranges, have a low GI. It is thought that the fibre in these foods slows down glucose absorption. Bread containing wholegrains, such as granary bread, has a lower GI than wholemeal bread, because the grain has been ground in wholemeal bread making it easier to digest.

The ripeness of a fruit and the cooking methods used also affect GI. For example, a green, unripe banana has a much lower GI than a ripe one; boiled new potatoes have a lower GI than baked or mashed potatoes. While fatty foods like chips, crisps and chocolate have lower GIs because their fat content slows down glucose absorption, they are best kept to a minimum because eating a lot of these will lead to weight gain.

Eating regularly also helps to stabilise blood glucose levels. Snacking on low-GI foods in between meals, such as oatcakes with cottage cheese or peanut butter (with no added sugar), berries, apples, oranges, or a handful of nuts or seeds, can help you avoid blood sugar peaks and troughs.

13. Power up with protein

Eating a little protein together with unrefined carbohydrates at each meal also helps to balance the blood sugar, as well as boost your brain's ability to deal with stress; protein slows down the rate at which glucose is released into the bloodstream and carbohydrate foods help the brain to absorb the tryptophan it contains. Tryptophan is an amino acid the body uses to make serotonin, a type of brain chemical known as a neurotransmitter. Neurotransmitters carry messages between nerve cells in the brain, and low levels of serotonin are associated with feeling stressed and anxious.

Protein foods that are good sources of tryptophan include turkey, chicken, fish, eggs, dairy foods, nuts, seeds, beans, oats, lentils and wholegrains. These foods also supply other amino acids such as tyrosine, lysine and arginine, which help the body to deal with stress by boosting serotonin levels, providing the raw materials for other neurotransmitters and regulating stress hormones.

14. Eat healthy fats

Fats have various important roles in the body, including ensuring the brain and immune system work properly; there is evidence that including the right types of fat in your diet can both help your body to cope with stress and reduce the harmful effects stress has on the body.

There are four main types of fat in the foods we eat:

Saturated – found mainly in animal products, e.g. red meat, butter and full-fat dairy products. These are solid at room temperature and are thought to raise harmful low-density lipoproteins (LDL) cholesterol, cause atherosclerosis (hardening of the arteries) and make our brain cells less flexible. They are also thought to make it harder for the brain to use polyunsaturated fats.

Polyunsaturated – essential fatty acids (EFAs) – found in fish, vegetable oils, nuts and seeds. These play a vital role in healthy brain function. The fats and oils we eat are broken down into fatty acids. Some fatty acids can be made by the body from other substances, but polyunsaturated fatty acids can't be produced in the body, so they have to be obtained from food – hence they are known as essential fatty acids (EFAs).

There are two main types of EFAs – omega-3, found in oily fish, nuts, seeds, and some plant seed oils, such as flax oil and rapeseed oil; and omega-6, found mainly in plant seed oils such as sunflower oil, corn oil and meat. Both omega-3 and omega-6 fatty acids are needed for the brain to function properly.

Trans (partially hydrogenated fats) – found in some margarines and processed foods, such as biscuits, pies and cakes. These are formed when liquid vegetable oils are turned into solid fats, through a process known as hydrogenation. If intake of EFAs is low and intake of trans fats is high, trans fats may replace EFAs in the brain, with detrimental effects on the way it functions.

Monounsaturated (omega-9) – found in olive oil, rapeseed oil, avocados, nuts and seeds. These lower LDL cholesterol, are anti-inflammatory and also have a role in brain function.

Get the balance right

Getting the right balance between the two types of EFAs is important. Too much omega-6 can hamper the body's ability to break down omega-3 fats and can exacerbate stress-related changes in the immune response that trigger inflammatory conditions such as eczema, asthma, psoriasis, rheumatoid arthritis and heart disease. Research suggests that omega-3 fats reduce the inflammatory response to stress. It's also thought they help the body adapt to stress by moderating adrenaline levels.

UK diets tend to contain too much omega-6, because many processed foods, cooking oils and margarines contain corn oil and sunflower oil – a ratio of omega-3 to omega-6 of around 1:10 instead of 1:3. So to counteract the negative effects stress has on your immune system you should aim to eat more foods containing omega-3 oils and fewer containing omega-6 oils. There are two types of omega-3 fatty acids:

- **Long chain** – found in oily fish, such as sardines, pilchards, mackerel, herring, salmon and fresh (not tinned) tuna. Aim to eat at least two portions a week.

- **Short chain** – found in flaxseed oil, rapeseed oil, pumpkin seeds, sunflower seeds, almonds, walnuts, wholegrains, wheatgerm and soya beans. Aim to eat up to two tablespoons of nuts (around 30g) and a tablespoon (15g) of seeds daily.

Tip: Sprinkle seeds and chopped nuts on your breakfast cereal and on salads; add seeds to sandwich fillings; use flaxseed or rapeseed oil as a salad dressing and in cooking.

Enjoy a glass of wine

A study published in the American Journal of Clinical Nutrition in 2008 concluded that moderate wine drinking (see Action 22 – Moderate your alcohol intake) increases blood levels of omega-3 fats. It's thought that the antioxidants in both red and white wine help the body to absorb omega-3 fats.

How much fat should I have?

The current advice is that fats and oils should make up no more than a third of your daily calorie intake. This equates to around 70 g (5 tbsp) for women, of which no more than 20 g (1.5 tbsp) should be saturated fat, and 95 g (7 tbsp) for men, of which no more than 30 g (2 tbsp) should be saturated fats. To give you some idea of your daily intake, here is the approximate saturated fat content of an average portion of some everyday dishes:

- Cheese and pickle sandwich: 10 g

- Fish and chips: 5.2 g (cooked in vegetable oil) / 22.7 g (fried in dripping)

- Sunday roast dinner: 9 g–14 g

- Lasagne: 12 g

- Curry: 20 g

- Pizza (per slice) – pepperoni: 9 g; seafood: 3 g; vegetable: 5 g

15. Curb your salt intake

Prolonged stress can trigger salt cravings, as the adrenal glands become exhausted (adrenal fatigue) and unable to produce adrenaline and cortisol, which can affect salt levels. A high intake of salt is linked with various health problems, including high blood pressure, coronary heart disease, stroke, stomach cancer, osteoporosis, kidney problems and stomach ulcers. Current guidelines suggest we eat no more than 6 g of salt daily, so satisfying a salt craving could easily push your daily intake beyond this level. Here is the salt content of some common foods:

Food	Salt content
Packet of crisps	0.5 g
4 g serving of Marmite	0.5 g
50 g serving of salted peanuts	0.7 g
100 ml serving of gravy (made with gravy powder)	1 g
400 g can of soup	3 g
Pre-packed sandwich	Up to 4 g
400 g tin of regular baked beans	5 g
Bacon sandwich	5.3 g

The best way to curb your salt intake is to eat meals prepared from fresh ingredients, cooked at home, using little or no salt. To avoid having to reach for the salt cellar to add flavour to meals, use black pepper, herbs, garlic, ginger and chillies to season your cooking. Squeeze lemon juice over fish and seafood to enhance their flavour.

When you haven't got time to cook from scratch, check food labels for the salt content. Be aware, however, that these can be misleading, as many food manufacturers give the sodium content, which has to be multiplied by 2.5 to work out the amount of salt. Also the sodium or salt content per 100 g is often given, which again entails arithmetic to calculate the total amount in a serving of the product.

Products listing any of the following in their ingredients are likely to be high in salt:

 Brine

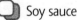 Garlic salt

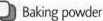 Onion salt

Soy sauce

Baking powder

Baking soda

Sodium and compound of sodium, e.g. monosodium glutamate, disodium phosphate

16. Eat ACE foods

Stress hormones such as cortisol can both lower immunity, raising the risk of colds and other infections, and over-activate it, triggering inflammation and autoimmune disorders like rheumatoid arthritis. The antioxidant vitamins A, C and E have a normalising effect, boosting immunity, and dampening down inflammation and autoimmune conditions.

Antioxidants are so-called because they protect the brain and the body from damage from free radicals (oxidative stress) by neutralising them. Free radicals are chemicals the body produces when it uses oxygen, and in reaction to infection, stress, exposure to sunlight and pollutants such as cigarette smoke, chemicals and food additives. They can cause damage to healthy cells and inflammation, a response by the immune system to protect the body from invasion by foreign substances. Symptoms include redness, heat, swelling and pain. Chronic inflammation happens when the immune system is overactive over a prolonged period of time and is blamed for various conditions, including allergies and autoimmune disorders. Autoimmune disorders are due to the immune system mistaking normal body tissues for 'the enemy' and attacking them. Below is an overview of the specific properties of each antioxidant and the foods that supply them.

Vitamin A is believed to protect the brain from oxidative stress and help maintain memory when under stress; it also boosts the immune system. It comes in two forms – as retinol and beta carotene. Retinol is found in animal products such as liver, fish liver oils, egg yolks, whole milk, cheese and butter. Beta carotene is found in plants – especially in yellow and orange fruits and vegetables, such as carrots, sweet potatoes, butternut squash, cantaloupe melons, orange and yellow peppers, and apricots. Note: Too much retinol can be harmful, so don't take a fish liver oil supplement with a multivitamin. Pregnant women in particular need to be careful, as excess retinol can cause birth defects. Beta carotene, however, is not toxic.

> ### Tip: Roast vegetables in olive oil
>
> To gain the most benefit from vegetables like carrots, peppers and sweet potatoes, roast them in a healthy fat, such as olive oil. Roasting softens the cell walls, making the beta carotene easier to digest, and adding fat helps the body to absorb it.

Vitamin C is involved in the production of noradrenaline and boosts immunity. Found in fruit and vegetables – especially citrus fruits, blackcurrants, berries, peppers (especially red), tomatoes, broccoli, potatoes, peas and cabbage. Vitamin C is also found in useful amounts in calf, lamb, beef and chicken livers.

Vitamin E is thought to protect the brain in particular from free-radical damage. Found in nuts, seeds, avocados, sweet potatoes, olive oil and wheatgerm.

17. Boost your B vitamins

When you are under stress your body's requirements for the B vitamins shoot up. All B vitamins are involved in the control of tryptophan, the precursor to serotonin. Vitamin B1 (thiamine) helps to produce energy from glucose and a lack of it is linked to irritability. Vitamin B3 (niacin) plays a part in the production of neurotransmitters. Vitamin B5 (pantothenic acid) is used to produce stress hormones.

Vitamin B6 (pyridoxine) is needed by the body to produce both serotonin and gamma-aminobutyric acid (GABA), another calming neurotransmitter that counteracts the effects of stress hormones; it is also needed for a healthy immune system. Both vitamin B9 (folic acid) and vitamin B12 (cobalamin) are involved in the production of SAMe – a chemical the body uses to make neurotransmitters, such as serotonin. Insufficient biotin (a B vitamin which, confusingly, is sometimes referred to as vitamin H) has been linked with panic attacks and low mood.

A balanced diet containing meat (including liver and kidneys), fish, eggs, dairy foods, wholegrains, vegetables – including green leafy vegetables, beetroot and mushrooms – citrus fruits, beans, peas, nuts, seeds and wheatgerm should supply enough B vitamins for most people's needs. If you're a vegan, eat a lot of processed foods or are under a lot of stress, you could be short of B vitamins and may benefit from taking a vitamin B complex supplement (see Chapter 6).

18. Value vitamin D

Vitamin D deficiency may make you more susceptible to stress because it's linked to low serotonin levels and poor immunity. It is thought to balance immune function and help to prevent autoimmune disorders. This vitamin also helps the body to absorb calcium, which plays a part in your ability to deal with stress (see below). A three-month trial at Queen Charlotte's & Chelsea Hospital, London, reported that eating a calcium and vitamin D-rich diet reduced premenstrual syndrome (PMS) symptoms, including irritability and fatigue, by about a third.

The best food sources of vitamin D are oily fish and liver – decent amounts can also be found in butter, milk, eggs, fortified margarines, cereals and powdered milk. However, we get around eighty per cent of our vitamin D from the sun; the skin produces a form of it following exposure to sunlight. This might explain why getting outdoors on a sunny day makes us feel happier and more relaxed. Many people in the UK are thought to be short of Vitamin D due to a lack of sunshine – especially in winter when the sun's rays aren't strong enough. Exposing the skin on the face and arms to thirty minutes of sunlight daily (without suncream) should provide enough vitamin D for most people. If you are fair skinned and burn easily, expose your skin for ten minutes at a time, three times a day.

Tip: Eat dishes with tomato-based sauces

Protect your skin from the damaging effects of the sun by eating dishes with tomato-based sauces. Research suggests that lycopene, an antioxidant in tomatoes that protects the plant from sunlight, may do the same for us. Cooking tomatoes releases the lycopene from the cell walls, making it easier to absorb. Guavas, pink grapefruits and watermelons also contain lycopene.

Remember, however, that overexposure to the sun's rays has been linked to skin cancer, so make sure you apply a suncream with a minimum sun protection factor (SPF) of 30 if you stay in the sun for longer than thirty minutes.

The recommended daily intake of vitamin D is between 10 and 15 micrograms (400–600 international units); however, nutritional therapists like Patrick Holford recommend at least twice this amount, 30 micrograms (1,200 international units) daily; two roll-mop herrings or four canned pilchards provide around this amount. For vegans, mushrooms are the main food source.

Supplementation is recommended if you can't get outdoors. If you take a fish liver oil supplement, avoid taking a multivitamin tablet as well, as vitamin D is fat-soluble, which means any excess is stored in the liver and fatty tissues; high levels can be harmful (see Action 43 – Benefit from supplements) and may even cause low mood.

19. Mind your minerals

Minerals are essential nutrients that your body and brain need in tiny amounts in order to function properly. Below is an overview of the minerals thought to be necessary for a healthy nervous system that is able to cope with stress.

Calcium and magnesium
Calcium and magnesium are often known as 'nature's tranquilisers'. Calcium is involved in the transmission of nerve impulses, hence a deficiency is linked with an inability to relax, nervous tension, irritability and insomnia. The richest sources of calcium are dairy foods – especially low-fat milk, reduced-fat hard cheese, Parmesan, Edam and yogurt. Tinned sardines are also a good source – provided you eat the bones. Good non-animal calcium providers include black molasses, almonds, seeds, tofu, soya, seaweed, dried figs, dates,

dried apricots, oats, Brazil nuts, watercress, leeks, parsnips, lentils, beans, and green leafy vegetables such as kale and purple broccoli.

Tip: Sprinkle a little vinegar

To help your body absorb the calcium they contain, sprinkle leafy green vegetables with a little ordinary vinegar. Drinking a tablespoon of cider vinegar and honey in warm water once or twice a day is also recommended for promoting calcium absorption. Vinegar is also good for keeping blood sugar levels steady because it slows down glucose absorption from food.

'Good' bacteria – probiotics such as lactobacillus – seem to enhance calcium absorption. There are various probiotic foods and drinks available, such as natural live bio-yogurts, Yakult and Activia. Prebiotic foods such as onions, tomatoes, leeks, garlic, cucumber, celery and bananas feed and promote the growth of probiotics in the gut, and also help. Remember calcium is also found in water – especially in hard water areas and some bottled waters.

Note: It's recommended that your daily calcium intake doesn't exceed more than 2,000–2,500 mg. A higher intake may interfere with the absorption of other minerals, such as iron, and could lead to other problems.

Magnesium is involved in the metabolism of the B vitamins and essential fatty acids, and has an important role in the absorption of calcium. It is also needed for the release of energy from foods, and for the proper function of nerves and muscles. A lack of magnesium can lead to raised cortisol levels, irritability, nervousness, low mood and insomnia. The Food Doctor Ian Marber describes magnesium as a 'fantastic relaxant' that 'enables your body to deal more effectively with stress', adding, 'so if your mind is working overtime then this is the mineral for you'. Your magnesium levels may be low if you are stressed, or if you eat a lot of sugary foods.

To make sure you get enough magnesium in your diet, eat plenty of dark-green leafy vegetables (such as spinach, broccoli and kale), seafood, tomato puree, nuts, seeds, wholegrains (including cereals like All-Bran and Bran Flakes), beans (including baked beans), peas, potatoes, oats and yeast extract. Avoid drinking too much alcohol as it can interfere with magnesium absorption (see Action 22 – Moderate your alcohol intake). Fizzy drinks are also best avoided, because the phosphates they contain also affect magnesium absorption.

Tip: take an Epsom salt bath

You can also soak up magnesium through your skin by adding one or two cups of Epsom salts to the bath as it fills. This is a great way to soothe tense aching muscles.

Chromium

Chromium helps to keep the blood sugar steady by working with insulin to remove excess glucose from the blood; we've talked about how peaks and troughs in blood sugar levels can affect your ability to deal with stress. Good sources of chromium include meat, wholegrains like oats and wholemeal bread, lentils and spices.

Selenium

Stress is thought to increase the need for the trace mineral selenium. Research published in *The Lancet* in 2000 reported that a shortage of selenium is linked with irritability, anxiety and low mood. Selenium is thought to affect the way neurotransmitters function and is needed for normal immune function. Selenium-rich foods include wholegrains, Brazil nuts, cashew nuts, wheatgerm, eggs, seafood (especially tuna, crab, oysters and lobster), meat (including kidneys and poultry), garlic, mushrooms and brewer's yeast.

Zinc

Stress increases your requirements for zinc. This mineral is involved in the production of neurotransmitters and is needed for normal immune function. A lack of zinc in the diet has been linked with anxiety and confusion, as well as a lack of concentration and motivation. Nuts, seeds, meat, eggs, seafood (mussels, prawns, sardines and oysters), beans, peas, mushrooms, broccoli, squash, spinach, kiwi and blackberries are all good sources of zinc.

Kitchen cupboard de-stressers

Did you know that some of the herbs, spices and fruits in your kitchen have de-stressing properties?

Basil booster – this pungent herb is believed to relieve stress and boost mood. To benefit, add torn basil leaves to pastas and salads.

Chilli calmer – eating chillies is thought to encourage the release of relaxing endorphins.

Lemon soother – drinking freshly squeezed lemon juice in hot water counteracts the effects of stress, according to Japanese researchers. The active ingredient is linalool – one of the substances responsible for the distinctive smell of lemons. If you find the taste too tart, sweeten with honey.

Rosemary relaxer – this aromatic herb is thought to calm and boost mood and memory. Try adding fresh rosemary spikes to stews and roasted vegetables.

Tarragon tranquiliser – this aniseed-flavoured herb is said to have calming, sedative properties. Its delicate flavour complements fish and chicken dishes.

Vanilla chiller – vanilla is believed to have a calming effect. Use it to enhance the flavour of cakes and desserts. Use dried vanilla pods or pure vanilla extract, as opposed to artificial vanilla flavouring.

20. Drink plenty of water

Your whole body – including your brain – needs sufficient water to function properly; research suggests that dehydration raises levels of the stress hormone cortisol. Experts recommend 1.5–2.5 litres of water daily; this may sound like a lot, but remember foods like fruit and vegetables have a high water content and therefore contribute to your daily intake. Also, tea and coffee can be counted as part of your fluid intake (they still contribute fluid, despite having a slight diuretic effect); however, they contain caffeine, so it's advisable not to drink too much, or to drink de-caffeinated versions instead.

21. Cut the caffeine

When under stress people often drink a lot of coffee for the stimulant effects of the caffeine it contains. If you drink coffee in moderation it can boost your mood and improve your alertness and concentration, because it induces the alarm stage of the stress response in the body – i.e. adrenaline and cortisol are released. However, if you regularly drink too much you are, in effect, producing the resistance and exhaustion stages of stress in your body and are likely to be jittery, anxious and unable to switch off – especially at bedtime; you may also experience raised blood pressure and increased heart rate. Caffeine can also be addictive because once the effects wear off your body craves more to give you another boost.

So if you consume a lot of caffeinated drinks and foods, such as coffee, strong tea, cola and chocolate, you might want to consider reducing your intake. The caffeine content of tea and coffee can vary quite widely, depending on the brand, how much coffee/tea is used and how long it is left to brew etc. It's hard to say how much caffeine is too much, as sensitivity to it varies from one person to another; however, most experts advise a daily limit of no more than 300 mg.

Herbal teas, redbush (rooibos) tea and decaffeinated coffee or tea make good alternatives to regular coffee and tea. Aim to wean yourself off coffee gradually to avoid withdrawal symptoms like headaches and anxiety.

Caffeine content of drinks/foods

Drink/food	Caffeine content
Tea (mug)	55–140 mg
Instant coffee (cup)	54 mg (on average)
Ground coffee (cup)	105 mg (on average)
Cocoa (cup)	5 mg (on average)
50 g plain chocolate	Up to 50 mg
50 g milk chocolate	25 mg (on average)

Herbal teas

Handy tip: use a coffee cafetière to make your herbal teas quickly and easily. Place the herbs in the cafetière, then add boiling water. Replace the lid and leave to brew for a couple of minutes, then press down the plunger and pour.

22. Moderate your alcohol intake

When you are feeling stressed you might feel tempted to self-medicate with alcohol, because it quickly makes you feel more relaxed. A UK survey by a health charity of more than 1,000 adults in 2006 reported that 34 per cent of men and 26 per cent of women viewed having an alcoholic drink as a way of helping them to feel less stressed.

However, if you are feeling stressed you should consider limiting your alcohol intake, because drinking excessively usually makes it worse; over-consumption of alcohol depletes various vitamins and minerals, including those that are needed for a healthy nervous system, such as B vitamins, calcium, zinc and magnesium and amino acids, like tryptophan. As we've already seen, deficiencies in these nutrients affect our ability to deal with stress and lead to irritability, mood swings, insomnia and other psychological problems.

Alcohol also temporarily boosts levels of the neurotransmitters that enable us to deal with stress, such as gamma-aminobutyric acid (GABA) and serotonin; however, when the effects wear off you may be left feeling jittery and anxious, because it also stimulates the release of adrenaline and has a depressant effect that can exacerbate a low mood. Drinking alcohol when under stress can also increase the amount of fatty deposits around the heart. Alcohol can disrupt your sleep patterns too: see Action 29 – Sleep more soundly.

Recommended safe weekly alcohol limits:

Women: 14 units
Men: 21 units
One unit roughly equals:
One small (125 ml) glass of wine; half a pint of beer or lager; one small glass of sherry or port; one single measure of spirits.

To learn more visit www.drinkaware.co.uk.

Note: Current recommendations are that men should not regularly drink more than three to four units daily and women no more than two to three units a day. Also, drinkers should have at least two drink-free days each week to give the liver a chance to rest and repair.

The de-stress diet

In a nutshell, the de-stress diet is a balanced, wholesome diet that contains wholegrains, oily fish, meat including poultry, low-fat dairy products, fresh fruit and vegetables, legumes (beans, peas and lentils), nuts, seeds, olive oil and plenty of water, to supply all the nutrients you need to enable your mind and body to cope with whatever life throws at you.

Cooking a healthy meal needn't take a long time. Try roasting vegetables such as peppers, tomatoes, onions and courgettes in a little olive oil with garlic, chilli and herbs. Add to cooked wholewheat pasta and stir in a low-fat cream alternative or a little more olive oil. You could add tuna, or a little Parmesan for added protein. Stir-fries only take minutes to prepare and cook. Broths and casseroles are easy to make – you can do other jobs once they're on the hob or in the oven. For extra speed, substitute frozen vegetables for fresh.

For more recipe ideas see the recipe section at the end of the book.

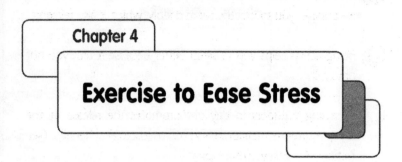

Chapter 4

Exercise to Ease Stress

When you are under pressure it is easy to forget to exercise, yet research suggests that being physically active can help to both prevent and ease stress. In 2008 a study in the *British Journal of Sports Medicine* concluded that any type of daily physical activity was associated with lower levels of stress. Researchers asked 19,842 men and women in Scotland how much exercise, and what type, they did every week. They also questioned them about their state of mind. The results suggested that walking and even domestic chores like housework and gardening reduced stress levels and boosted mood.

There are several reasons why exercise can help:

Exercise uses up the 'fight or flight' hormones adrenaline and cortisol, which are released during the stress response.

During physical activity the body releases the 'happy' hormone serotonin, as well as endorphins, which act like natural tranquilisers, relieving stress and boosting mood.

Exercise takes your mind off the stresses and strains of everyday life, while focusing on your chosen activity encourages you to live in the moment.

Moving around warms and loosens tense muscles and encourages you to breathe more deeply, which is also relaxing.

Being active helps you to sleep better because it tires you out physically.

Exercising outdoors in daylight promotes the release of the 'sleep' hormone melatonin and has psychological benefits (see Action 24 – Enjoy ecotherapy).

Studies show that people who take regular exercise have higher self-esteem – possibly because they feel more confident about their bodies and have a sense of achievement. Going to an exercise class or a gym is also a great way to meet other people with similar interests, which can have a beneficial effect on your emotional health. However, you don't have to go to the gym to lead an active lifestyle; this chapter also suggests other easy ways to incorporate exercise into your everyday routine. We look at activities such as walking, outdoor exercise, Pilates, swimming, t'ai chi and yoga, and the stress-relieving benefits they offer.

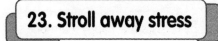

23. Stroll away stress

Walking is a great way to improve your mental health and general fitness. An eight-year study in the US suggested that menopausal women who walked for 40 minutes at least five times a week experienced less stress, anxiety and depression than less active women.

Even if you are really busy it is possible to fit more walking into your daily routine. There are the obvious strategies, such as parking your car further from the office, or the shops, or getting off the bus or train one stop earlier. Other easy ways to walk more include:

- Park your car at the top of a multi-storey car park, then use the stairs down and back up.

- Get up from your desk and walk around regularly.

- Use the stairs rather than the lift.

- Take a 15-minute walk during your lunch break, instead of sitting at your desk.

- Walk to your colleagues' desks to pass on information instead of emailing them.

- Walk to the water dispenser every hour or two for a refill – your brain will benefit from the exercise and the increased hydration.

- Make trips to the kitchen to make drinks for colleagues.

- Walk your dog every day – if you don't have one, offer to walk a neighbour's.

Benefit from walkies!
Research suggests dog owners take more exercise and are fitter than gym users. This is probably down to the fact they have to exercise their pets 'come rain or shine'. On average a dog walker clocks up 676 miles a year compared with just 468 miles for a gym-goer. Dog walkers generally have lower blood pressure and their heart rates

return to their resting rate faster than gym users. So, if you want to enjoy the benefits of your own canine personal fitness trainer, buy a dog, or offer to walk a neighbour's!

Pet power

Did you know that stroking your pet dog or cat could help to cut your stress levels? Studies show that the body stops producing the stress hormones cortisol and adrenaline, and the heart rate drops when you fuss over a pet.

---

24. Enjoy ecotherapy

Research by Essex University for the mental health charity Mind, published in 2007, concluded that ecotherapy (engaging with nature) has both mental and physical health benefits; ninety-four per cent of the 108 people who took part in 'green exercise', such as gardening, walking, cycling and conservation work, reported feeling more relaxed and having improved self-esteem. Following these findings Mind called for ecotherapy – especially 'green exercise' – to be more widely recognised as an effective treatment for mental distress. As a result, GPs in some areas of the UK are referring people suffering from stress, depression or anxiety to 'green gyms', which offer the opportunity to participate in conservation projects.

In 2004 research by Japan's National Land Afforestation Promotion found that a walk in woodland lowered blood pressure and heart rate, and boosted the immune system. It also reported that people who stopped to admire a pleasant woodland view for twenty minutes had 13 per cent less cortisol in their bloodstream. The Japanese call this calming, grounding effect of trees *shinrin-yoku*, meaning 'forest bathing'. Experts claim the higher levels of negative ions near areas with running water, trees and mountains may be involved. Others say the effectiveness of ecotherapy is down to 'biophilia' – the belief that we all have an innate affinity with nature and that our disconnection from it causes stress and mental health problems.

Aim at spending some time outdoors in a 'green space' – such as a garden, a park or woodland – each day. Even just a few minutes spent outdoors can be beneficial; research at Essex University in 2009 suggested that spending five minutes in a green space cut stress levels. To enjoy the most benefit, include some 'green exercise' such as walking, cycling or gardening; being outdoors gives the additional benefits that result from exposure to sunlight, such as increased vitamin D levels (see Action 18 – Value vitamin D) and sounder sleep (see Action 29 – Sleep more soundly).

25. Practise Pilates

Pilates is a low-impact exercise programme devised by the gymnast Joseph H. Pilates to tone the abdominal (core) muscles, and stretch and strengthen the whole body. It promotes correct posture, which helps to boost your mood and prevent muscular tension and pain, as well as deep, controlled breathing, which can help to relieve stress. In her book, *Pilates for Every Body*, the US fitness programme presenter Denise Austin claims this form of exercise 'helps you feel mentally and emotionally balanced, calm and refreshed'.

Pilates can be practised at home, as there are various instructional DVDs available, but it is probably best to join a class at first, to ensure you adopt the correct posture and perform the exercises correctly; most leisure centres and health clubs now offer Pilates classes. The Body Control Pilates Association provides details of qualified instructors (see Directory).

26. Swim away stress

According to the Chief Medical Officer's report on the health benefits of physical activity, published in 2004, swimming has psychological as well as physical benefits; it confirms that being in a pool can 'take you away from it all'. Many people find being in water relaxing, probably because it supports the weight of the body. Also, when you are swimming you have to concentrate on your breathing, rhythm and stroke, which takes your mind off your worries and encourages you to live in the moment. Swimming in the sea is especially relaxing, because it is another form of 'green exercise'. When you visit your local public swimming baths, if possible choose times when it isn't too busy, such as during weekdays or perhaps weekend evenings, to avoid being jostled or interrupted. To improve your swimming technique visit www.swimfit.com, a website that offers an online coaching programme.

27. Chill out with t'ai chi

T'ai chi, described as a 'moving meditation', is an ancient Chinese non-combative martial art that promotes both mental and physical well-being. The movements are slow and controlled, helping to improve strength, flexibility, posture and balance. The discipline is viewed as part of traditional Chinese medicine because it aims to promote the smooth flow of *qi* ('life energy') through channels in the body, known as meridians. There is some evidence that t'ai chi can relax the muscles and help to reduce mental and emotional stress.

It is possible to learn t'ai chi at home using an instructional DVD (see Directory) but it is probably better to learn how to perform the movements correctly initially by joining a class – for details of classes near you visit www.taichifinder.co.uk.

28. Say yes to yoga

The word 'yoga' comes from the Sanskrit word *yuj*, which means union. Yoga *asanas* (postures) and *pranayama* (breathing exercises) are designed to unite the body, mind and soul. Hatha yoga is a slow, gentle form of exercise, which not only strengthens the joints and muscles, increasing flexibility and mobility, but also loosens tight muscles, relieves stress and induces calm. The word 'hatha' means 'balance', from the Sanskrit words '*ha*' meaning sun and '*tha*' meaning moon; the postures and breathing exercises have balancing effects on the body and mind.

In a German study in 2005, the stress levels of 24 women who described themselves as 'emotionally distressed' were measured using the Cohen Perceived Stress Scale; all of the women were found to have higher than normal scores for perceived stress. Sixteen of the women attended two ninety-minute yoga classes each week for three months, while the eight women in the control group kept to their normal activities and agreed not to begin an exercise or stress-reduction programme during the study. At the end of the study the women in the yoga group showed much bigger improvements than those of the women in the control group. The study also found that the cortisol levels of the yoga group fell after each class.

All yoga poses relieve stress by releasing tension that has built up in the body; below is a breathing exercise and four *asanas* you might want to try:

Alternate nostril breathing *(nadi shodhana)*
This yoga breathing exercise helps to promote calm and clarity of mind.

1. Press your right nostril closed with your right thumb. Inhale slowly through your left nostril to the count of four.

2. Hold your breath for as long as is comfortable. Release your right nostril and block your left nostril with your right index finger.

3. Exhale slowly through your right nostril. Now inhale through your right nostril to the count of four. Hold your breath. Release your left nostril, exhaling.

4. Repeat this cycle five to ten times.

Standing forward bend *(pada hasthasana)*
You can perform this basic stretch as a warm-up at the beginning of your yoga session, or whenever you need to release tension from your neck, shoulders and back.

1. Stand with your feet together, your arms at your sides.

2. Inhaling, stretch your arms above your head, extending your body as far as you can, from the base of your spine to your fingertips. Hold for a few seconds.

3. Exhaling, bend forwards. Grasp the backs of your legs as far down as you can, pushing your forehead towards your knees. Hold for a few seconds.

4. Repeat up to five times.

The tree (*vrksasana*)

This *asana* calms the mind and improves balance.

1. Stand with your feet slightly apart, your knees straight and your arms and shoulders relaxed.

2. Exhaling, put your left foot on the inside of your right thigh, as high up as you can, with the toes pointing downwards.

3. Inhaling, stretch your arms to the sides, palms facing down.

4. Exhaling, put your hands together in the prayer position.

5. Raise your arms above your head keeping your hands in the prayer position. To keep your balance, focus on a point in front of you and keep on breathing in and out, slowly and rhythmically. Stay in this pose for about one minute.

6. Repeat on the other side.

The cobra (bhujangasana)

This posture is especially good for easing tension in the neck and back muscles.

1. Lie on your front with your legs together and your forehead resting on the floor.

2. Place your hands beneath your shoulders, palms down and fingers pointing towards each other.

3. Inhaling, tilt your head backwards and slowly raise your trunk, pushing down with your hands.

4. Arch your back slowly, bringing your trunk as far back as you can without straining.

5. Hold the pose for a few seconds.

6. Exhale slowly, gradually uncurling your spine as you lower your trunk back down to the floor.

7. Relax for a few seconds in the original position. Repeat two more times.

The cat (bidalasana)

This *asana* loosens the muscles in the shoulders and upper back and improves breathing.

1. Kneel on all fours, with your head tilted backwards, and your arms and back straight. Your hands should be directly beneath your shoulders and your knees directly beneath your hips.

2. Exhaling, arch your back as high as you can, pulling your tummy in and curling your head inwards. Hold for a few seconds.

3. Inhaling, hollow your back and lift your head, looking upwards. Hold again. Repeat sequence five times.

Learn yoga

The best and probably the most enjoyable way to learn yoga is to attend classes run by a qualified teacher. To find one near you, go to the British Wheel of Yoga's website – www.bwy.org.uk. Or, if you'd prefer to teach yourself at home, visit www.abc-of-yoga.com – a site which shows you how to achieve the various postures, using animated clips. You can buy CD and MP3 hatha yoga class downloads, suitable for all levels and abilities, and download a free taster session at www.yoga2hear.co.uk. You can also find yoga information, products and guidance at www.yoga-abode.com.

Safe yoga

When practising yoga at home, always proceed slowly. Avoid forcing your body into position and stop if you feel any discomfort. Wear lightweight, loose clothing to enable you to move freely, and no footwear, as yoga is best performed barefoot. Use a non-slip mat if the floor is slippery. Don't try inverted postures if you have a neck or back problem, or have high blood pressure, heart disease or circulatory problems. If in doubt, consult your GP first.

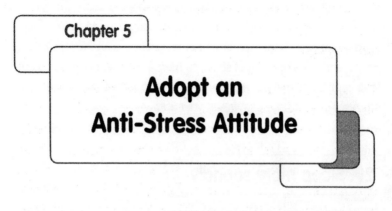

Chapter 5

Adopt an Anti-Stress Attitude

'Stress is perceived in the mind, suffered in the human spirit, experienced via the emotions, expressed in behaviour, and held in the body.'

Anonymous

The stress response starts in your brain. If you perceive an event to be a threat or a challenge your brain immediately sends messages to your nervous, hormonal and immune systems, and the stress response is triggered. Studies have shown that when people learn how to control their emotions the amount of the stress hormone cortisol released into the bloodstream in response to potentially stressful situations is greatly reduced.

In this chapter you will learn how to change the way you think, to reduce the amount of stress you experience. Stress often underlies sleep problems, and a lack of sleep can trigger the stress response and negatively affect your mood and attitude towards life, so there are tips to help you sleep more soundly. There are techniques from cognitive behavioural therapy (CBT) to help you replace negative thoughts and attitudes about yourself and the world around you with more positive ones. You will learn how to solve problems effectively, find out how living in the present can make life less stressful and discover how to be more assertive. Anger management strategies to help you avoid the harmful effects of losing your temper are also included.

You will learn how self-acceptance and being true to yourself can help you feel more relaxed and at ease. Change is an inevitable part of life, and a major cause of stress, so there are tips to help you accept and cope with change, and to confront the fears that prevent you from making positive changes in your life.

29. Sleep more soundly

Stress is one of the main causes of sleep problems, because feeling wound up or worried makes it hard to fall asleep and stay asleep. Lack of sleep is a major stressor because during sleep part of the brain processes and stores information, while the brain cortex rests and recovers. Also, the body repairs tissue wear and tear, and produces growth and appetite-regulating hormones, as well as disease-fighting white blood cells. After just one night of poor sleep we are less able to cope with pressure and are more likely to be irritable, have poor concentration and short-term memory, and succumb to infections – all of which can contribute to a vicious cycle of stress and insomnia. Recent research also suggests that insomniacs have a four times greater risk of experiencing relationship problems and are twice as likely to have energy dips.

To sleep more soundly try these tips:

Get outdoors in daylight to stop the production of melatonin, the brain chemical that promotes sleep; this makes it easier for your body to release it at night, so you fall asleep more quickly and sleep more soundly. Blue light, which is light from a blue sky on a clear day, is thought to be the most beneficial.

Eat foods rich in tryptophan, an amino acid from which your body produces first serotonin and then the 'sleep' hormone melatonin. Tryptophan-rich foods include chicken, turkey, bananas, dates, rice, oats, wholegrain breads, cereals and dairy foods, which also contain calming calcium – which is why a glass of milk at bedtime can aid sleep.

Ensure you're neither too hungry nor too full when you go to bed, as both can promote wakefulness.

Avoid drinking coffee or cola, or eating chocolate after 4 p.m. – the stimulant effects of the caffeine they contain can last for hours. While tea has around half as much caffeine – about 50 mg per cup – it's best not to drink it near bedtime if you have sleep problems. Redbush (rooibos) or herbal teas, which are caffeine-free, make good alternatives.

Exercise raises your body temperature and metabolism, which fall a few hours later, encouraging sleep. Avoid exercising after 8 p.m., otherwise your body temperature could still be raised at bedtime, promoting wakefulness. Insufficient exercise can cause restlessness and difficulty sleeping.

Wind down before bedtime. Develop your own routine in the evening that allows you 'put the day to bed'. This might involve watching TV – if you find it relaxing – but avoid tuning in to anything that could prey on your mind later when you're trying to go to sleep and aim at switching the TV off at least half an hour before bed. Alternatively try reading or listening to music. Dim the lights to encourage your body to release sleep-inducing melatonin – a dimmer switch, lamp, or candles are ideal for this.

Enjoy a warm bath at bedtime. Your temperature rises with the warmth and then drops, helping you to fall asleep. The warmth can also help ease muscular and mental tension – especially if you add relaxing essential oils like lavender or chamomile.

Avoid drinking alcohol at bedtime. It might help you relax and drop off more quickly, but it also disrupts sleep patterns, so that you have less deep sleep. It is also a diuretic, so you are more likely to wake up to go to the toilet during the night.

If abstinence from alcohol doesn't help you sleep better, try a glass of Cabernet Sauvignon, Merlot or Chianti – these wines are made using melatonin-rich grape skins.

Make your bedroom as cosy and inviting as you can, to make bedtime a pleasure.

Keep your bedroom cool. Your brain tries to lower your body temperature at night to slow down your metabolism and aid sleep. A temperature of around 16°C is ideal.

Hang dark, heavy curtains, or wear an eye mask, to block the light. Darkness stimulates the pineal gland in the brain to produce melatonin.

Choose a mattress that gives you the right level of support; lie on your back and slip a hand beneath your lower back. There should be just enough room to fit your hand in the gap between your back and the mattress. If there's no gap, the mattress is too soft. A bed board under the mattress could help. If there's a lot of space, the mattress is too hard for you.

Pick a pillow that keeps your spine aligned with your neck. The best pillow depth for you depends on the width of your shoulders – if you have narrow shoulders choose a flatter pillow; if you have broad shoulders, you might need two pillows.

To help your brain associate your bedroom with sleep and sex only, banish TVs, computers, iPads and mobile phones. Watching TV, using a computer or other technology last thing at night can over-stimulate your brain, making it hard to switch off and fall asleep. Screens also emit bright light, which can affect the production of melatonin.

If mulling over problems or events taking place the next day prevents you from dropping off, try jotting down your concerns or a plan for the day ahead before you go to bed. If you find it hard to relax at bedtime you could try one of the meditation techniques outlined in Action 33 – Meditate.

If you wake during the night and start worrying about problems, try telling yourself firmly: 'You can't do anything about this now, so go to sleep and think about it tomorrow.'

Try this:
Imagine your worries are inside a helium balloon. Now picture letting go of the balloon and watching it, and your worries, float further and further away.

Only go to bed when you feel drowsy. If you don't fall asleep within about 20 minutes, get up and do something you find relaxing, like reading or listening to soothing music. Only return to bed when you feel sleepy, to help your brain associate your bed with sleep.

Finally, if you have problems falling or staying asleep try not to worry, as this will make you feel even more stressed and even less likely to drop off; instead bear in mind research suggests most people underestimate the amount of sleep they have had and can lose a few hours sleep now and again without experiencing too many problems.

30. Try the ABC of CBT

Cognitive behavioural therapy (CBT) is a type of psychotherapy that focuses on removing the negative thoughts and unhelpful behaviours that can lead to emotional issues including stress. It works on the underlying principle that your thoughts affect your feelings, your feelings affect your actions and your actions come full circle to affect your thoughts again. According to cognitive theory, many of us form negative beliefs about ourselves as a result of our experiences during childhood and early adulthood, e.g. being bullied at school, parents divorcing, failing an exam etc., and that these take root in our minds until they become automatic. Behavioural theory is based on the belief that behaviour is a learned response that is also a reaction to past experiences. CBT is based on both principles.

According to CBT your feelings aren't facts – they are just your perception of an event or situation. In other words, an event or situation is only stressful if you think it is. Your perception of events in your life and how you respond to them is down to the filters through which you view them. These filters include your personality, values, beliefs and attitudes, which have been shaped by your genetics, upbringing, past experiences, lifestyle and culture. However, it is possible to change your perception of an event and your subsequent behaviour, simply by changing your beliefs about yourself and situations.

Try the ABC approach next time you're feeling stressed:

Activator – note down the situation that triggered your stress, e.g. moving house.

Beliefs – list your thoughts about the situation, e.g. 'I can't cope', 'I don't like change'.

Consequences of A plus B – record your feelings and actions, e.g. worried, apprehensive, procrastination.

Dispute your negative thoughts; that is, identify alternative, positive ways of viewing the situation, e.g. 'I've moved house before and I coped very well', 'I'm looking forward to settling in my lovely new home', 'this move will be a change for the better'.

Effective new approaches – choose new, helpful thoughts and behaviours, e.g. 'I'll make a list of what needs to be done', 'I'll ask my family and friends to help me pack'.

If you follow this formula each time you face difficulties, you will gradually build a more positive image of yourself and your ability to cope with whatever life throws at you. This will give you the confidence to find effective solutions and reduce the amount of stress you experience.

31. Solve problems effectively

According to Eckhart Tolle, author of *The Power of Now*, there are no problems, only situations that either have to be dealt with, or accepted and left alone. While this might sound over-simplistic, it is a useful way to approach life's difficulties. Much the same message is offered by the 'Serenity Prayer', which advocates accepting the things we can't change, having the courage to change the things we can, and having the wisdom to know the difference.

Tolle argues that if you spend too much time mulling over issues, you end up being overwhelmed by them or with thoughts of what you will do, instead of taking appropriate action to resolve them *now*. Research at the University of Missouri in 2007 seems to back up this philosophy. Psychologists found that when teenage girls talked about their problems excessively it made them seem much more serious than they were, and kept the girls stuck in a negative frame of mind, which led to stress and low mood.

When you focus your energies on what you can do now to solve a problem, it no longer seems insurmountable. Even taking the smallest step towards a solution today can make you feel better and more in control of your situation, which in turn reduces stress levels.

Try this:

1. Write down the problem.

2. Identify actions you can take towards resolving the problem *now*. For example, if you wrote: 'I'm worried about money', identify ways you could improve your finances. Could you earn more money either by working more hours or by generating

a second income from something you could do in your spare time, such as babysitting, dog-walking, or direct selling, e.g. become an Avon representative? Could you spend less by managing your money better (see Action 8 – Take control of your spending)? If you can't cope with your debts, could you speak to your creditors, or contact a helpful organisation like Citizens Advice or National Debtline to ask for advice?

3. 'I never have enough time to do everything' – identify ways you could save time, e.g. by saying 'no' to things you don't need to do, delegating tasks and adopting easier ways to do things, such as speed-cleaning your home and simplifying your beauty routine – for more ideas see Chapter 2 – Simplify Your Life.

4. 'I've got relationship problems' – try to identify the source of the discord and what you can do about it. If it is down to lack of time for each other, think of ways you could make more time. If you have children, could you hire a babysitter to enable you to have regular 'date nights'? If you and your partner can't resolve your issues you might consider contacting Relate for relationship counselling.

5. Ask yourself: What advice would I give to a friend with this problem? It is usually easier to come up with answers to other people's problems because we are detached from them.

6. If there is nothing you can do about the problem now, accept it and do something to distract yourself from it, e.g. do some chores, go for a walk, or meet a friend for coffee – anything that stops you dwelling on the issue.

32. Live in the moment

'As you walk, eat and travel, be where you are. Otherwise you will miss most of your life.'

Buddha

As a small child you probably found it easy to live in the moment, because you weren't burdened by your past and hadn't yet developed a fear of the future. As a result you were able to enjoy life as it unfolded, minute by minute. Once you reached adulthood, however, it's likely you started dwelling on the past and worrying about what might happen in the future, both of which increase your stress levels unnecessarily.

Enjoy life now

It's much easier to cope with everyday life when you focus on the 'here and now', because you can concentrate fully on the task in hand, whereas worrying about the past and future can hamper your performance. Living in the moment is known as mindfulness. A review by the US National Academy of Science suggested that living in this way led to less stress and boosted the immune system.

When you live in the present you should find your life more enjoyable and less stressful, because instead of doing things on autopilot, all of your senses are focused on what you're doing. For example, imagine going for a walk in a beautiful park while being so preoccupied with worries about the future, or regrets about the past, that you aren't even aware of your surroundings. Now imagine going for the same walk, but this time noticing the beauty of the trees and plants around you, hearing the sound of birdsong and inhaling the scents and aromas, and think how much more pleasurable and relaxing it would be. On a more practical level, if you focus on the task in hand at work, instead of worrying about other jobs you need to do, you are likely to complete it more quickly and efficiently. If you don't have a lot of time to spend with your family, focusing completely on them when you are together, rather than thinking about, or doing, other things at the same time, will be far more rewarding for everyone

Living in the present is a skill that can be learned. Don't worry if you find it difficult at first – whenever you notice your mind wandering bring it back to the here and now. Yoga involves focusing on your breathing and your body as you carry out different postures, and is a good way to practice living in the moment. Taking part in a sport or doing something you find absorbing, like cooking a meal, painting a picture, knitting or sewing, can also bring you back to the present. Keeping a daily diary might help, too, because it encourages you to think about what has happened in your life today.

Try this:

Start by focusing on your breathing – notice the rise and fall of your chest as you breathe in and out.

Identify any tension in your body – tighten the affected muscle, then relax it.

If you're eating, concentrate on the sight, smell, taste and texture of your food – don't watch TV or read at the same time.

If you're having a conversation, actively listen to what the other person is saying, instead of letting your mind wander.

◯ If you're doing a chore like washing up, or ironing, focus fully on what you are doing.

◯ If you go outdoors, use all of your senses to take in the sights, sounds and smells around you as you walk.

Don't worry

'Unease, anxiety, tension, stress, worry – all types of fear – are caused by too much future, and not enough presence.'
Eckhart Tolle, *The Power of Now*

Living in the present means focusing your energy on dealing with real situations, instead of wasting it worrying about those that may never happen; so rather than fretting about what could go wrong at an impending event, such as a meeting, job interview or exam, take practical steps to prepare for it now, so that you feel more confident and in control. If you feel overwhelmed by the size of a task, rather than worrying about it, break it down into achievable steps.

It also means not trying to predict the future; how many times have you lain awake at night thinking of the worst possible outcomes to a current situation only to find a few days/weeks/months down the line things turned out far better than you expected and your agonising was unnecessary? Worrying about events that haven't happened triggers the stress response, because your body can't tell the difference between what has happened in reality and what you imagine happening. For example, if you worry about being made redundant and not being able to pay your bills, your body will release stress hormones, even if you don't actually lose your job.

Although it's hard not to think about the things that could go wrong in your life, it's better for your mental health if you can make a conscious effort not to worry about things that may never happen. It's also important to accept that not everything in life is easy and to put things in perspective.

Try this:
List some situations you've worried about in the past. Beside each one write the outcome you feared most. Now mark each outcome with a tick or a cross to indicate whether or not it happened in reality. You should find:

a) Most, if not all, of your concerns didn't materialise and/or:

b) Even if your worst nightmare did happen, you eventually came to terms with it and moved on.

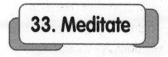

33. Meditate

Like living in the moment, meditation involves focusing your mind on a particular activity, thought, or object and disregarding any distractions.

Clinical studies have shown that mediating regularly induces deep physical and mental relaxation, reversing the effects of the body's fight or flight responses to stress. A review of 20 studies on the effects of meditation on health concluded the technique could help people cope with epilepsy, premenstrual syndrome (PMS), menopausal symptoms, autoimmune disease and anxiety.

Below are five different types of meditation: the first involves focusing on your breathing; the second involves visualising a relaxing scene; the third involves focusing on a particular statement (affirmation); the fourth meditation involves deep breathing while concentrating on a selected colour; and the final one involves tensing and relaxing your muscles, as you breathe in and out.

Bo-Tau

With each breath we take, oxygen is absorbed into the blood to enable the production of energy necessary for every function of the body. When we're stressed our breathing tends to be fast and shallow – which leads to a drop in the level of calming carbon dioxide in our bloodstream. This can make us even more stressed and cause muscular tension in the neck, shoulders and upper back. Slow, deep breathing appears to slow the heart rate, increase production of calming alpha brainwaves, relax muscles, relieve tension, and trigger the release of 'happy hormones' serotonin and dopamine.

Focusing on your breathing also helps to take your mind off your worries and is a simple form of meditation. So the next time you're stressed or anxious, take control of your breathing. The slow-breathing technique outlined below, known as Bo-Tau (breath optimised transformational unblocking), was devised by neuropsychologist Dr David Lewis.

1. Ensure you are sitting or lying comfortably.

2. Close your eyes and start focusing on your breathing.

3. Inhale slowly and deeply through your nose for five seconds, allowing your stomach to expand. Hold for five seconds.

4. Exhale slowly for ten seconds, as you gradually pull your stomach in.

5. Whenever a passing thought distracts you, simply return to focusing on your breathing.

Visualise your favourite retreat

Visualisation enables you to escape from everyday stresses and strains, and can be done whenever you have a few spare minutes.

1. Find a comfortable place to sit or lie and close your eyes.

2. Focus on breathing in and out deeply as in the previous exercise.

3. Next picture your favourite retreat – for example, a golden beach with blue skies, turquoise sea and lush palm trees, or maybe a country garden filled with roses and honeysuckle.

4. Now use all of your senses to explore your retreat – feel the warmth of the sun on your face and body, hear the crash and roar of the waves, smell the sweet perfume of the roses and honeysuckle.

5. Enjoy the scene until you feel ready to return to reality.

6. Breathe in and out slowly and deeply. When you are ready, open your eyes.

For more information on mindfulness take a look at the Mental Health Foundation's Be Mindful campaign www.bemindful.co.uk.

Affirm and relax

Using affirmations (also known as mantras) to help you relax is another form of meditation. An affirmation is a positive statement that describes what you want to achieve or feel in the present tense with the idea that your subconscious mind will accept it as a reality. Here are some examples of affirmations for reducing stress and promoting relaxation: 'I am relaxed'; 'I am calm'; 'I am at peace'; 'My muscles are relaxed'.

1. Choose an affirmation that suggests relaxation to you.

2. Sit quietly and close your eyes.

3. Breathe in and out slowly, and deeply, as in the previous two exercises.

4. Repeat your affirmation on each out-breath.

Colour breathing

This is another variation of deep, relaxing breathing that involves concentrating on a particular colour as you breathe. There is a strong link between colour and emotions; certain colours and colour combinations can make us feel cold, warm, happy or sad, and the colour of our surroundings can have a big effect on our mental well-being. Blue has been shown to aid relaxation and green is thought to relieve nervous tension. This might be because these are the colours of nature, i.e. the blue sky and green plants and trees, and scientists believe we have a natural affinity with nature.

1. Follow the deep-breathing exercise above.

2. On each in-breath imagine your body is filling up with the colour blue or green.

3. Note how each colour makes you feel, so that you can choose the one that relaxes you the most whenever you feel stressed.

Practise muscle relaxation

When you feel stressed and anxious you're likely to tense your muscles, which makes you feel even more stressed. When you release the tension in your muscles you automatically feel more relaxed.

Try this muscle relaxation sequence before or after other meditations, or whenever you feel stressed.

Take a deep breath in through your nose, then tense the muscles in your face by clenching your teeth and screwing up your eyes tightly. Relax and breathe out through your mouth.

Take a deep breath in through your nose, then raise your shoulder muscles, tense them for a few seconds and then relax. Drop your shoulders and release the tension as you breathe out through your mouth.

Take a deep breath in through your nose, then clench your fists and tense the muscles in your arms, hold for a few seconds then release and breathe out through your mouth.

Next, breathe in through your nose, tighten the muscles in your buttocks and legs, including the thighs and calves, hold, then release as you breathe out through your mouth.

Finally, breathe in through your nose, clench your toes and tense your feet, hold, then release and breathe out.

34. Turn a negative into a positive

When difficult situations do arise, changing your attitude towards them can reduce the stress they cause, because it's how you interpret the event, not the event itself that triggers your emotional response. When something bad happens, after initially thinking how terrible the situation is, try to find something good about it if you possibly can. Look for positive solutions to your problems, or view them as opportunities for personal growth. For example, even though being made redundant might seem like a negative event initially it can turn into a catalyst for positive change in the long run, as people often find they are forced to retrain and start a new, exciting career doing something they really enjoy,

Try this:
Think of a difficult situation you experienced in the past. Now list any benefits you may have gained from the situation in the long term. For example, after the heartache and trauma you initially had to face, getting divorced may have eventually enabled you to develop independence and self-reliance, or begin a new, happier relationship; the lifestyle changes you had to make in order to overcome financial difficulties may have gradually helped you to learn how to manage on less money and appreciate the simple things in life more; a year or two on from dealing with a serious illness you may have realised you are stronger and more resilient than you previously thought.

Lighten up!

Lightening up and seeing the funny side of things, even when life delivers you a blow or you experience minor mishaps, could reduce your risk of the health problems associated with stress. Laughter has been shown to cut levels of the stress hormones cortisol and adrenaline, boost levels of the 'happy hormone' serotonin and release pain-relieving endorphins. It also relaxes the muscles, lowers blood pressure and boosts the immune system. Watching your favourite comedies and comedians, and being around people who make you laugh, could also help you cope with adversity. Or try visiting www.laughlab.co.uk or www.ahajokes.com whenever you feel like a good giggle!

35. Reach out to others

Often when you feel tense or overloaded the last thing you want to do is see other people. But there's evidence that seeing family and friends regularly helps to reduce stress, so it's worth making an effort to get out and meet people, even when you don't feel like it. Talking to other people can help to take your mind off your problems, or even help you find solutions, whereas sitting at home alone just gives you more time to dwell on things.

Being in a happy, long-term relationship has been shown to help buffer the effects of stress; in 2007 a study of 400 nurses working in hospitals in Yorkshire found that those who were happily married or in a stable relationship were less affected by the pressures of their job. Those who were widowed experienced more stress and divorcees suffered the most stress. Researchers thought the married nurses benefited simply from having someone to offload their woes to at the end of a stressful working day.

Nurture your relationships

When we are really busy and stressed our personal relationships are one of the first things to suffer. Often our working lives and domestic commitments take precedence over spending quality time with our partners, family and friends. The first obvious step is to look for ways to make time for your relationships. Chapter 2 – Simplify Your Life suggests ways to save time in your everyday life.

Is your relationship a cause of stress?

If you're not receiving the support you need from your long-term partner, you might benefit from giving your relationship an overhaul. Below is a brief overview of the key areas you might want to consider:

1. **Communication** – being able to talk about your thoughts and feelings is vital for a healthy relationship. Problems can escalate if you bottle up how you really feel. Ask your partner if you can both set aside regular time to discuss your expectations and feelings. Choose your time for talking carefully – offloading your issues when one or both of you have just walked through the door after a tough day at work might not be the best time. Take turns to talk and then listen to each other. Try not to criticise or attach blame (see Action 37 – Assert yourself for tips on communicating effectively without being aggressive

or antagonising). Women should remember that men are often wary of talking about emotions, but they do like to solve problems; so the best way to get them on board is to ask them to help you find an answer.

2. **Appreciation** – try not to take your partner for granted. Remind yourself that you are lucky to have a good partner. Say 'thank you' every day for the things they do for you: not only does it make them feel appreciated, but it also makes them more likely to want to do more for you! Research has shown that people need five positive experiences to get rid of the memory of one negative one. So aim to dish out five positive comments for every negative one you make.

3. **Caring** – show your partner that you care – a hug and a kiss or even a cup of tea can make them feel loved. Hugging is a great stress reliever because it releases the 'cuddle' hormone oxytocin in both the giver and the receiver; oxytocin has anti-stress effects, including lowering cortisol levels and blood pressure.

4. **Sharing** – make sure domestic chores are shared out fairly between you; otherwise it is likely to cause tension and resentment in your relationship. Make a list of tasks, then discuss with your partner who should do what.

Shared interests can help to bind you both together and give you something to talk about other than work and your domestic commitments. Shared time together is the lifeblood of any relationship so try to set aside time together every day – even it is just to catch up on each other's day, go for a walk or watch a TV programme together. However, there needs to be a balance – having some separate friends and interests can help to keep your relationship fresh.

36. Manage your anger

When people are stressed they are more likely to have a 'short fuse' and get angry about trivial things that wouldn't normally bother them. At the time they feel their anger is justified, but often, when looking back, they realise they have overreacted. Anger is, in effect, an extreme stress response. As well as being a sign of stress, anger can also raise stress levels. Recent research published in the *International Journal of Psychophysiology* reported that not only does blood pressure rise during a bout of anger, but it also rises whenever we think about the event that triggered it – even days later. Numerous studies suggest that angry, hostile people are more prone to heart disease.

The first obvious step to managing anger is to cut the amount of stress in your life by following the advice in this book, so that you don't overreact to irritations in the first place. On the other hand, if you are annoyed or upset about something, it's important that you express these feelings; repressing them can cause stress, anxiety and depression. If you find yourself in a situation that makes you angry, the techniques below should help you take control of your emotions and express your anger in a healthier way.

1. Recognise that you can choose to be calm in trying or difficult situations.

2. Take a deep breath and count to ten, or walk away temporarily if you can – this helps to counteract the stress response and defuse the situation, making you less likely to say or do something you will regret later.

3. Accept that other people will act according to their rules and values, rather than yours.

4. Accept that other people have a right to have and express their own views – even if they differ from your own.

5. Show empathy – try to see things from the other person's perspective, rather than just your own. You might realise they are not deliberately setting out to annoy or upset you.

6. Communicate your feelings calmly, avoiding shouting or suggesting blame, e.g. say: 'I feel angry when you…' instead of 'You make me angry when you…'

7. Detoxify the situation with an apology, e.g. 'I didn't mean to upset you.'

8. Try to raise your tolerance of minor mishaps and delays. Ask yourself: is this situation really worth getting angry about?

9. Take exercise to release tension. Physical activity uses up the stress hormones and energy your anger has generated.

10. Let go of resentment. Resentment is the result of holding on to anger and does you, the bearer, harm, rather than the person or situation that caused it.

Expressing how you feel appropriately can help you avoid feeling stressed or angry. Below are some tips on how to be assertive.

37. Practise assertiveness

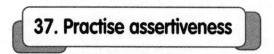 Do you often hide your true feelings instead of expressing them?

Do you inadvertently give in to others so that you don't hurt or upset them, or to gain their approval, and only realise what you have done in hindsight?

◯ Do you regularly allow others to manipulate you into doing things you don't want to do?

◯ Do you bottle up feelings until you eventually explode with anger?

◯ Do you act in an aggressive or intimidating way when you are angry?

If you answered 'yes' to any or all of these questions you may benefit from improving your assertiveness skills. Being assertive involves saying what you want, feel and need, and standing up for your rights, calmly and confidently, without being aggressive or hurting others.

The Assertiveness Bill of Rights

1. I have the right to express my feelings.
2. I have the right to express my beliefs and opinions.
3. I have the right to say 'no'.
4. I have the right to change my mind.
5. I have the right to say 'I don't understand'.
6. I have the right to be myself.
7. I have the right to decline responsibility for other people's problems.
8. I have the right to make reasonable requests of other people.
9. I have the right to set my own priorities.
10. I have the right to be listened to.

The following techniques will help you to express your emotions and remain in control of your life, doing things because you want to, rather than to please other people, which will help you avoid unnecessary stress and anger.

 Choose the right time and place to talk.

Maintain eye contact but don't stare, as the other person may find this threatening.

Speak calmly, clearly and firmly – avoid shouting.

Think carefully about what you want to say before you speak.

Aim to be concise and to the point, rather than rambling.

Take ownership of your thoughts, feelings and behaviour by saying 'I' rather than 'we', 'you' or 'it'. Rather than saying 'You make me angry', try something like 'I feel angry when you…' – this is less antagonising to the other person.

When you have a choice whether or not to do something, say 'I won't' or 'I am not' rather than 'I can't' to show that you've made an active decision, rather than suggesting something, or someone, has stopped you. Use 'I want to' instead of 'I have to', and 'I could', rather than 'I should', to demonstrate you have a choice. For example: 'I am not going out tonight', rather than 'I can't go out tonight', or 'I could go out tonight, but I want to stay in'.

If you feel your needs aren't being considered, state what you want, repeating it until the other person shows they've heard and understood what you've said.

When making a request, identify exactly what it is you want and what you're prepared to settle for. Choose positive, assertive words, as outlined above. For example: 'I would like you to help me tidy the kitchen. I'd really appreciate it if you could empty the dishwasher.'

When refusing a request, give the reason or reasons why without apologising. For example: 'I'm not visiting you today, because I've been really busy at work all week and have a lot of chores to catch up on.'

If you disagree with someone, tell them using the word 'I'. Explain why you disagree, but acknowledge the other person's right to have a different viewpoint. For example: 'I don't agree that the service in that shop is poor – we waited a long time to get served last time because it was very busy, but I can understand why you think that.'

38. Accept yourself

Do you constantly compare yourself, for example your appearance or your achievements, to those of other people and then beat yourself up for not being slim/pretty/handsome or clever/rich/successful enough? This kind of thinking can lead to discontent and unnecessary stress, because it makes you feel you must constantly strive to improve yourself or your life in some way to be happy. So you start thinking: 'I'll be happy when I've lost weight/got a promotion/met a new partner/bought a better car/bought a new house.'

According to leading psychologists and spiritual teachers, you can only be happy when you stop trying to be perfect, and accept and like yourself as you are now. You don't have to achieve impossibly high standards to earn your own and other people's love and respect. There will always be someone who is cleverer/prettier/slimmer/richer/more successful than you, but there will never be another you, with your unique mix of abilities, weaknesses, successes and failures. If you choose to accept and value yourself, warts and all, you'll realise you are good enough as you are now and instantly feel more relaxed and at ease with yourself.

Try this:

Next time you start beating yourself up about some aspect of your life, with negative self-talk like 'I'm a failure', 'I'm useless', 'I'm stupid', imagine you have a kind, caring, friend who knows all your strengths and weaknesses but still loves and accepts you as you are. This friend understands that who you are and what you do is often down to things that are beyond your control, including your past experiences, your upbringing, your personality and your current circumstances, and that everyone fails sometimes – it's part of the risk we take when we try new things. Now write down what you think your friend would say to you about your perceived imperfections, e.g. 'You are/look great the way you are', 'You're doing your best' and 'You've achieved a lot'. Whenever you find yourself being self-critical, think what a good friend would say.

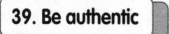

39. Be authentic

'Your time is limited, so don't waste it living someone else's life.'
Steve Jobs, co-founder of Apple

Being authentic means behaving in a way that meets your own needs, rather than simply to please others. This might sound selfish, but psychologists have found that the more authentic people are, the happier and more fulfilled they are likely to be. Not allowing yourself to be who you really are can lead to stress and unhappiness, and this will have a negative impact on the lives of people around you. Quite simply, if you are happy and fulfilled you will be nicer for others to be around.

Many of us spend our lives trying to be someone we're not – perhaps doing a job we don't enjoy because it pays well, or because our parents wanted us to follow a particular career path. Life is too short to spend it doing things you don't enjoy. Not allowing yourself to be who you really are can lead to stress and unhappiness. For example, if you love being outdoors, working in an office for 40 hours a week might not be the best career choice. Being your authentic self means living a life that reflects your values and passions, and utilises your particular strengths and talents.

Does your life reflect who you are?

'Life is so much easier when you know who you are.'
        Fiona Harrold, *Reinvent Yourself: Seven Steps to a New You*

Complete the questions below to check how authentic you are.

1. Are you living your values?
Your values are the things that are most important to you. Identify the five things you value most. The list below might give you some ideas:

 Family

 Relationships

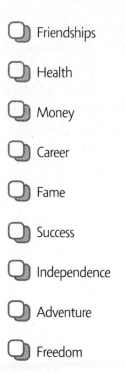

Friendships

Health

Money

Career

Fame

Success

Independence

Adventure

Freedom

Now think about each of your values and ask yourself: What is it about this value that is important to me? For example, if you chose 'family' or 'relationships', the value underpinning it might be 'love'. If you chose 'money', the value underpinning it might be 'feeling secure'.

Now check whether you are living your values. If you're not, how could you? With these two examples this might mean spending more time with the people you love, or looking at ways to earn more money or reduce your outgoings to improve your financial security.

2. Are you playing to your strengths?

Your strengths are your positive personality traits. Note down what you consider are your main strengths. The list below might give you some ideas:

Creativity

 Kindness

Leadership

Curiosity

Empathy

Loyalty

Team working

Fairness

Optimism

Persistence

Bravery

Organising

Ask: Do I play to my strengths at work and at home?

If you answered 'no': Identify ways you could use your strengths more. For example, if you're a good organiser, but hate cooking, could you do more of the organising at home, e.g. manage the household budget, arrange holidays, write the shopping list etc. and ask your partner to do more of the cooking? Could you use your organisational skills more in your job, e.g. set and meet deadlines, initiate ideas, delegate tasks, arrange meetings? If not, could you look for a job that involves using organisational skills?

3. Are you using and developing your talents?

'... have the courage to follow your heart and intuition. They somehow already know what you truly want to become.'

Steve Jobs, co-founder of Apple

Your talents are the tasks and activities you have a natural aptitude for. The most successful people from all walks of life throughout history have excelled by concentrating on what they are good at. Being aware of and using your natural talents boosts your self-esteem, and motivates you to achieve more and be successful, whereas forcing yourself to do things you aren't good at can sap your confidence because it forces you to focus on your inadequacies. Would people at the top of their chosen field, such as Jamie Oliver, Tiger Woods, J. K. Rowling, Kate Winslet, Joan Collins and Richard Branson, have been as successful if they hadn't used their innate talents?

Everyone has a natural ability. You might be extraordinarily good at mental arithmetic, writing, languages, public speaking, teaching, cooking, gardening, interior design, singing or acting. You might excel at sports, music, or arts and crafts. If you can find the time to do the things you are really good at you are more likely to fulfil your potential and be at peace with yourself.

If you haven't already recognised your talents, try this:

1. List anything you find really easy to do well. The tasks that we do almost effortlessly are the ones we have a natural talent for.

2. Next note down your passions. What really interests you? What did you love to do when you were younger? What excites and inspires you?

3. Now check both lists and identify any common activities. These are the areas where you are most likely to excel in life and find fulfilment. Once you have identified where your natural abilities lie, ask: am I using and developing my talents at work or at home?

If you answered 'no': Identify ways you could start using and developing your talents. For example, if you're good at maths, but lack the formal qualifications you need to enable you to get a job that involves numbers, perhaps you could enrol on a course in accounting at college, or train as a financial adviser?

If your passion is fashion you might decide to find a job in a boutique or enrol on a dressmaking class in your spare time.

If you are good with animals you might find a part-time job that involves working with them, for example, in a vet's or a boarding kennel, or you might keep pets, perhaps breeding and showing them.

These might sound like obvious choices, but it's surprising how many people spend their lives doing jobs they don't particularly enjoy and allow their spare time to be gobbled up with chores or passive pastimes like watching TV, when they could be doing the things they love most and excel at. If you are naturally good at something, you might find a way to develop it from a hobby to a career.

40. Appreciate what you have

It is human nature to take the good things in our lives for granted – a loving partner, good health, a fulfilling job, supportive friends, a lovely home, plenty of food to eat... the list could go on and on.

The trouble is, when we have these things around us all the time we stop noticing and appreciating them; instead we tend to focus on what we lack, which leaves us feeling dissatisfied and unhappy. Research suggests that people who notice and express gratitude for the good things in their lives are happier and more optimistic than those who complain about what they don't have. Being thankful for what you have brings peace of mind and true prosperity, whereas always wanting more raises your stress levels.

Try this:
Before you go to sleep tonight think of at least three good things that happened today. It could be something as simple as a smile from a stranger, a glorious sunny day, reading a good book, eating a delicious meal, or something more profound like the love of your partner, or the thoughtfulness of a friend.

41. Deal with change

Change is an inevitable part of life – without it we would become bored and lack opportunities to grow and stretch ourselves. However, as we've already mentioned in Chapter 1, change is also a major cause of stress – especially when it is due to circumstances beyond our control, e.g. redundancy or bereavement. Yet resisting change because we're frightened to let go of something that is no longer right for us can also lead to long-term stress. Many of us stay put in a bad situation because we fear the unknown.

For example, we may cling on to an unhappy relationship because we're afraid we won't meet anyone else and will end up alone, or stay in a job we hate because we can't face looking for alternative employment. In situations like these having the courage to walk away means we are saying 'yes' to new opportunities and experiences in our life, and hopefully a happier, less stressful life. It's only by leaving a bad relationship or unhappy work situation that you can find a new and better one. The key to dealing with change is to develop resilience. Resilience is basically the ability to bounce back after setbacks. It is a quality that anyone can develop at any stage in their life, and it can help you to turn adversity into an advantage and a threat into an opportunity.

Develop resilience

Top tips for developing resilience and dealing with change:

1. Accept that change happens.
2. Cultivate optimism – believe that things will improve.
3. Take control of your situation, rather than seeing yourself as a victim.
4. Be adaptable and willing to learn new things.
5. Take positive action to solve problems.

Cope with loss positively

If you are coping with divorce, bereavement, or redundancy, give yourself time to grieve your loss. As you gradually come to terms with what has happened you will experience a lot of different emotions, including shock, disbelief, sadness, hurt, anger, confusion, guilt and fear – and not necessarily in that order. Talk about your feelings, or write them down, and cry if you need to – bottling up your emotions can cause depression in the long term. It's only by experiencing the painful reality of your loss that you can begin to pick up the pieces and move forward with your life. Make plans for a positive future; set yourself achievable goals and do something every day to make them a reality. Look after yourself – eat healthily, take exercise and pamper yourself a little.

As you work your way through the grieving process, while creating a new life for yourself, you should find that you gradually come to terms with your loss and find a way to move on.

Case study

When Maria was in her early 40s and finishing a degree, her partner passed away suddenly. She says: 'Initially I was numb with shock; then I felt angry: why had this happened to me? I soon realised I could either keep on going over the past and feeling sad and angry, or I could focus on the present and building a new future. So although I gave myself time to grieve every day, I also concentrated on completing a degree, so that I could get the job I needed to support myself and my new future.'

Connect with your spirituality

For some people, it is helpful to connect with a spiritual force to find peace and happiness through prayer, meditation, or even being close to nature. Knowing there is a part of you that remains unchanged no matter what and that the external world is always subject to change can help you to cope with difficult times, as you realise they will eventually pass. For more information about connecting with your spiritual self go to www.eckharttolle.com.

42. Overcome fear

Fear can be paralysing and can prevent us from making the changes we need to make in our lives to be happier and less stressed. Many of us stay in our comfort zone rather than confront our fears. According to Susan Jeffers, author of *Feel the Fear and Do it Anyway,* it is no good waiting until the fear goes away before you take that first step. She says the only way to lose your fear is to go out and do whatever it is you are afraid of doing. Eventually you will lose your fear, before moving on to the next situation you find scary. If you stay stuck in your comfort zone rather than taking a risk, you will always be afraid. Doing things when you are frightened of doing them requires courage – the payoff is that you get to expand your horizons and develop your self-confidence.

Try this:
Identify something small you could do that takes you out of your comfort zone. For instance, if the idea of complaining to a stranger scares you, take a faulty or unsuitable item back to a shop and ask for a refund. If you usually wait for your friends outside because you feel embarrassed about walking into a restaurant on your own, arrange to meet them inside.

Once you have tackled minor fears like these you will feel more confident about confronting bigger challenges.

Deal with panic attacks

Panic attacks are a sign of stress and can be triggered by a traumatic event such as bereavement or divorce, or a major life change, like having children, or moving house.

A panic attack is a rapid build-up of overwhelming fear and can include several of these symptoms: a pounding, irregular heartbeat; chest pains; breathing difficulties; dizziness; feeling faint; nausea; a choking sensation; sweating; trembling; fear of losing control/blacking out/dying; a sense of danger; or feelings of unreality.

Hyperventilation (over-breathing), caused by breathing too quickly, is often a feature of panic attacks; this disturbs the oxygen and carbon dioxide balance in the body, leaving you with too little carbon dioxide and too much oxygen, which causes the symptoms described above. Most panic attacks last for about two minutes, but they can sometimes last for up to an hour. Sufferers often become anxious in between attacks, because they worry about when the next one is going to happen.

Three simple ways to overcome hyperventilation

Next time you start over-breathing try one of these instant fixes:

1. Hold your breath for as long as you can without feeling uncomfortable – usually this is for 10–15 seconds. Repeat a few times if you can. This helps you to retain carbon dioxide.

2. Breathe in and out of a paper bag – this makes you re-inhale the carbon dioxide you have exhaled.

3. Go for a brisk walk or run while breathing in and out through your nose; this helps to tackle the tendency to over-breathe.

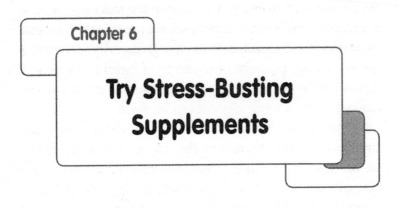

Chapter 6

Try Stress-Busting Supplements

This chapter looks at the various herbal, vitamin and mineral supplements commonly recommended for the relief of stress, outlining what each supplement is, what it does and how it works, as well as advice regarding its safe use.

If you find it hard to eat a balanced diet for whatever reason, supplements can help you safeguard against nutritional deficiencies. They are controversial, with some recent reports claiming that isolated substances don't provide the same benefits that nutrients found naturally in foods do. However, supplements can offer a convenient way to improve our diets and benefit from particular herbs, vitamins and minerals.

Do supplements work?

Often there is anecdotal evidence, but no, or insufficient, conclusive evidence that a supplement works. While there is a need to be cautious about unsupported claims, sometimes the lack of evidence is simply due to the fact that the research hasn't been done; even though the turnover in the herbal medicine sector is quite high, many individual manufacturers are unable to meet the high financial costs of clinical trials. So a lack of evidence to back up the use of a supplement doesn't necessarily mean it doesn't work, or isn't safe – but it is important to exercise some caution and make sure you only buy products from reputable companies. It is reassuring to know that the Medicines and Healthcare Products Regulatory Agency (MHRA) has recently tightened up the regulation of herbal medicines and supplements to help ensure their effectiveness, safety and quality (see below).

Another problem is that some herbal remedies have several active ingredients and this can make it difficult to identify which produce the beneficial effects. Also the quality of herbal medicines can vary quite a lot due to differences in plant species, the type of soil they are grown in and methods of extraction and storage etc. These variations can sometimes make it difficult to draw any firm conclusions about particular herbs.

Are supplements safe to use?

It is important to remember that just because something is termed 'natural' it is not necessarily harmless. Vitamins, minerals and herbs contain chemicals that have an effect on the body, just as drugs do.

Supplements fall under two categories – herbal medicines and food supplements – and are subject to legislation to help ensure the safety of the people who use them.

Regulation of herbal medicines

According to the MHRA, a herbal medicine is any medicinal product that contains one or more herbal substances as active ingredients, or one or more herbal preparations, or a combination of the two. Since April 2011, all herbal medicines have had to be registered under the Traditional Herbal Medicines Registration Scheme, or hold a product licence. Registered herbal medicines have to meet specific safety and quality standards and carry agreed indications for when they should be used. Licensed herbal medicines have to meet certain standards of safety, quality and effectiveness. For more information go to: www.mhra.gov.uk/howweregulate/medicines/herbalmedicines/index.htm.

Regulation of food supplements

Vitamin and mineral supplements are defined as food supplements and come under the EU Food Supplement Directive. This legislation aims to protect consumers from unsafe products by making sure all supplements are correctly labelled, and only contain permitted amounts of permitted vitamins and minerals. Manufacturers aren't allowed to make therapeutic claims about their vitamin and mineral supplements.

Find out more

MHRA provides a list of herbal products currently registered under the Traditional Herbal Medicines Registration Scheme, along with information sheets on their safe use. You can also report any adverse reactions from herbal remedies or supplements to the agency. Its contact details can be found in the Directory at the end of this book.

43. Benefit from supplements

Below is an overview of herbal, vitamin and mineral supplements, for which there is some evidence of effectiveness in the relief of stress, and that some people have found beneficial. They are available in various forms, including capsules, tablets and tinctures; you can grow some of the herbs mentioned in your own garden and use them to make herbal infusions, or you can buy them in teabag form. Related products are listed in the Useful Products section at the end of the book.

Ashwagandha
What it is: A plant that belongs to the pepper family and is grown in India and Africa. The root has been used in traditional Indian (ayurvedic) medicine for more than 2,000 years. Also known as *Withania somnifera*, winter cherry, or Indian ginseng.

What it does: Ashwagandha acts as an adaptogen, boosting endurance, stamina, brainpower and immunity, while reducing anxiety and promoting sleep. Traditionally believed to rejuvenate and extend life.

How it works: The active ingredients, withanolides, are thought to have sedative, antioxidant, and blood pressure- and heart rate-lowering properties.

Evidence it works: A study involving 39 people suffering from anxiety disorder in 2000 suggested that ashwagandha reduces anxiety; further research is needed, as the study was small and only lasted for six weeks. Animal studies suggest that ashwagandha improves sleeping patterns and brain function, boosts immunity during periods of stress and reduces cortisol levels; however, further human research is needed.

Safety: Thought to be safe when taken as directed.

Available as: Capsules (e.g. Pukka Organic Ashwagandha), tablets (e.g. Good 'N Natural Ashwagandha).

Eleuthero

What it is: Eleuthero is a plant native to south-eastern Russia, northern China, Korea and Japan. The root and rhizomes (underground stems) are the part of the plant used. It is also known as Siberian ginseng or Devil's shrub.

What it does: It increases stamina and energy, improves mental alertness, boosts immunity, and helps the body to avoid stress-related illness.

How it works: The active ingredients include eleutherosides and complex sugars thought to help moderate the stress response; it is thought there is a stress threshold below which eleuthero will raise the stress response and above which it will lower it. These active ingredients may also help the body produce energy.

Evidence it works: In a study involving 50 men and women, Polish researchers claimed that those taking eleuthero tincture three times a day for one month were fitter and had more stamina than those taking echinacea. In another study at the University of Iowa 96 people with chronic fatigue were given either eleuthero or a placebo. According to the researchers, those taking eleuthero reported less fatigue. When German researchers checked the immune function of 36 people before giving them 10 ml of eleuthero three times a day for four weeks, they reported it increased T-helper cells, which play a major role in the immune system. A German study published in the journal *Antiviral Research*, concluded that eleuthero has a 'strong antiviral' action.

Safety: Can occasionally cause diarrhoea initially and insomnia if taken too close to bedtime. Not recommended for people with high blood pressure. Take for six to eight weeks, followed by a two-week break as the beneficial effects reduce after eight weeks.

Available as: Tablets (e.g. Lifeplan Siberian Ginseng), capsules (e.g. Sibergin 2500 and Solgar Siberian Ginseng Extract) and liquid (e.g. Health Aid Siberian Ginseng Liquid).

Hops

What it is: A British climbing perennial plant. The part of the plant that is used is the flowers.

What they do: They act as a mild sedative, relieve stress and encourage sound sleep.

How they work: Hops have a sedative effect on the central nervous system, but the mechanism involved is not known.

Evidence it works: Dried hops have traditionally been used to treat anxiety, restlessness and insomnia. One study reported that hops and valerian combined promoted sound sleep. The German Commission E recommends hops for the relief of restlessness, anxiety and mood disorders.

Safety: No side effects have been reported, but hops can enhance the sedative effects of sedatives, sleeping tablets and alcohol and have a slightly depressant effect, so they are not recommended for people with depression.

Available as: A herbal tincture (e.g. G Baldwin & Co Hops Flowers and Dormeasan Valerian-Hops Oral Drops 50 ml) and tablets (e.g. Stressless and Kalms).

> The German Commission E is an expert committee in Germany that reviews herbal drugs and preparations from medicinal plants for their quality, safety and effectiveness.

L-lysine & L-arginine

What they are: L-lysine and L-arginine are amino acids involved in the production of neurotransmitters and regulation of stress hormone levels. Vegetarians and vegans may be short of L-lysine because vegetable and vegetable proteins contain very little.

What they do: They improve the ability to handle stress and relieve stress-induced anxiety.

How they work: L-lysine helps to increase serotonin levels by reducing its reabsorption into the nerve cells. Both L-lysine and L-arginine are thought to help balance levels of cortisol and adrenaline during times of stress.

Evidence they work: In a study in 2005 at the Slovak Academy of Sciences, 29 men suffering from anxiety were given either 3 g each of L-lysine and L-arginine daily or a placebo for ten days, before being asked to deliver a public speech. The results suggested that those taking the amino acids were able to handle pressure better than those taking the placebo. Another study of 108 healthy Japanese adults in 2007 claimed that those taking 2.64 g each of L-arginine and L-lysine every day for a week were less anxious in stressful situations.

Safety: L-lysine is generally safe, although high doses can cause gallstones. Don't take L-arginine if you are prone to cold sores, as it can trigger an outbreak. L-arginine can lower blood pressure, so don't take it if you have low blood pressure or you are taking a blood pressure-lowering medication (hypertensive). People with kidney or liver disease and pregnant or breastfeeding women should speak to their GP before taking an L-lysine or L-arginine supplement.

Available as: Tablets (e.g. Holland & Barrett L-Lysine 1,000 mg, Nature's Best Pure Lysine 500 mg and Solgar L-Arginine 500 mg Vegetable Capsules).

L-tyrosine

What it is: An amino acid used by the body to produce the neurotransmitter dopamine and the stress hormone adrenalin – which give you your 'get up and go'.

What it does: Helps to boost mental and physical performance when you are under stress.

How it works: It's thought that levels of dopamine and adrenaline fall when people are under stress. Supplementing with L-tyrosine when you are under extreme stress is thought to help replenish these chemicals.

Evidence it works: A small study in Holland in 1999, involving 21 cadets on a gruelling six-day combat training course, showed that those who took L-tyrosine performed better mentally than those who didn't. Another double-blind study found that L-tyrosine helped to prevent a decline in mental performance caused by sleep deprivation. Several controlled studies suggest that supplementing with L-tyrosine helps to boost mental performance in physically stressful situations such as extreme cold or noise.

Safety: If you suffer from a psychiatric condition, check with your doctor that it is safe for you to take before using.

Available as: Capsules (e.g. Holland & Barrett L-tyrosine 500 mg, Biovea L-tyrosine 500 mg).

Omega-3 Essential Fatty Acids (EFAs)

What they are: EFAs are fats the body needs for various functions, but can't produce itself. Omega-3 EFAs are found in oily fish, nuts, seeds and seed oils; if you don't eat these foods regularly a supplement may be beneficial.

What they do: Help the brain to work efficiently and normalise immune function during periods of stress.

How they work: The body obtains eicosapentaenoic acid (EPA) and docosahexaenoic acid (DHA), which brain cells need to function properly. DHA protects against stress-induced lowered immunity, and inflammatory and allergic conditions by preventing changes in the balance of cytokines (type of white blood cell).

Evidence they work: Various studies suggest that omega-3 fats moderate the effects of stress on the immune system. Double-blind, placebo-controlled research published in the *Nutrition Journal* in 2004, involving 45 university staff, concluded that supplementing the diet with fish oil – providing 1,500 mg of DHA and 360 mg of EPA daily for six weeks – reduced levels of perceived stress.

Safety: Omega-3 EFAs can interact with blood-thinning drugs, such as warfarin. The recommended daily amount for mental well-being is 1,000 mg of EPA/DHA; both fish oil and cod liver oil are good sources of EPA and DHA. Cod liver oil also contains vitamin D, which many people in the UK are deficient in (because the leading source is sunlight), and vitamin A. However, it is advisable not to take cod liver oil alongside a multivitamin, as any excess vitamin A and D is stored in the liver – too much of these vitamins can be harmful. Alternatively, if you are a vegetarian you could take flaxseed (also known as linseed) oil – but the body obtains less EPA/DHA from plant sources.

Available as: Oil and capsules (e.g. Pulse Omega-3 Pure Fish Oils).

Passion flower

What it is: Passion flower is a climbing shrub with purple and white flowers, native to South America and popular with gardeners in the UK. Both the flowers and leaves can be used and it is also known as passiflora.

What it does: It combats stress and calms an overactive mind.

How it works: The active ingredients, alkaloids, are mildly sedative, possibly because they enhance the effects of the neurotransmitter GABA.

Evidence it works: In 2010 a review into herbal supplements for anxiety by the Global Neuroscience Initiative Foundation, a mental health charity, concluded that passion flower is effective for the relief of anxiety.

Safety: Very rarely, passion flower may cause dizziness, confusion, heart problems and inflammation of blood vessels. Very rarely, there may be severe toxicity, even with normal doses. Do not take passion flower if you are pregnant or breastfeeding.

Available as: Tablets (e.g. RelaxHerb Passion Flower Extract 425 mg), liquid extract (e.g. Passiflora & Valerian Plus 50 ml) and tincture (e.g. G Baldwin & Co Organic Passiflora, Napiers Skullcap, Oat and Passionflower Compound).

Rhodiola rosea

What it is: Rhodiola rosea is an extract from the rhizome and root of the rhodiola plant, which grows in Scandinavia, Canada, Siberia and northern China. It's also known as golden root or Arctic root.

What it does: It relieves symptoms of stress, including fatigue and mild anxiety, and boosts concentration.

How it works: The active ingredients are rosavins, which act as adaptogens, raising tolerance of physical, mental and environmental stress by acting on the hypothalamus in the brain. They may also help to carry tryptophan and 5-hydroxytryptophan (5 HTP) to the brain.

Evidence it works: Several studies suggest that rhodiola rosea increases tolerance to stress. In 2000, a study of 40 students during exam time found that those taking rhodiola rosea had less mental fatigue and better physical fitness than those taking a placebo. In 2009, another study at Uppsala University in Sweden, involving 60 people with stress-related fatigue, suggested that those receiving rhodiola rosea had better concentration and lower levels of the stress hormone cortisol than those taking a placebo.

Safety: Do not take rhodiola rosea if you are pregnant, or suffer from kidney or liver problems.

Available as: Tablets (e.g. Vitano Rhodiola Rosea Root Extract 200 mg), capsules (e.g. Viridian Maximum Potency Rhodiola Rosea Root Extract 250 mg) and alcohol-free extract (e.g. Nature's Answer Rhodiola Root Alcohol Free Extract 30 ml).

Valerian

What it is: A tall fern-like plant with pink and white flowers, sometimes known as 'nature's valium'. The root is used in herbal medicine.

What it does: It may help to relieve stress, anxiety and stress-related muscle tension, as well as insomnia.

How it works: Valerian is thought to increase levels of the neurotransmitter GABA, which has a calming, tranquilising effect.

Evidence it works: Valerian is a traditional herbal remedy for stress and anxiety, and is approved by the German Commission E for use as a mild sedative. In a double-blind trial involving 48 adults, who were put in an experimental situation of social stress, valerian supplements reduced anxiety without causing sedation.

Safety: *Valeriana officinalis* is thought to be safe, but some other types of valerian may cause liver problems. Occasional side effects include drowsiness, mild headaches and nausea. Very rarely, it may cause nervousness and excitability. Pregnant or breastfeeding women shouldn't take valerian due to lack of information regarding safety. If you are taking prescribed medications be aware that valerian can interact with some, e.g. loperamide, a drug used to treat diarrhoea, and fluoxetine, an SSRI antidepressant, to cause delirium, so always speak to your GP or pharmacist first before taking it.

Available as: Tablets (e.g. Stressless, Kalms), liquid extract (e.g. Passiflora & Valerian Plus 50 ml) and tincture (e.g. Dormeasan Valerian-Hops Oral Drops 50 ml).

Vitamin B complex

What it is: Vitamin B complex, often known as 'the anti-stress vitamins', is a group of vitamins with several important roles in the body – including within the nervous and immune systems. You could be short of B vitamins if you eat a lot of processed foods, if you are a vegan, or if you are under a lot of stress.

What it does: Supports vital processes in the body, especially during times of stress.

How it works: B vitamins are involved in various processes that are important during times of stress, including the production of the calming neurotransmitters serotonin and GABA, maintaining a steady supply of glucose to the brain and releasing energy from cells.

Evidence it works: In a double-blind study in 2000, 80 healthy men aged between 18 and 42 were randomly assigned to receive a supplement containing vitamin B complex, vitamin C, calcium, zinc and magnesium or a placebo for 28 days. The multivitamin contained the following: thiamine (15 mg), riboflavin (15 mg), niacin (50 mg), pantothenic acid (23 mg), vitamin B6 (10 mg), biotin (150 micrograms), folic acid (400 micrograms), vitamin B12 (10 micrograms), vitamin C (500 mg), calcium (100 mg), magnesium (100 mg) and zinc (10 mg). Compared with the placebo group, the multivitamin group experienced consistent and statistically significant reductions in perceived stress, as determined by questionnaires measuring psychological state. This group also tended to rate themselves as less tired and better able to concentrate.

Safety: Taking B vitamins is generally safe. However, you should take a supplement containing no more than 100 mg of vitamin B6 – higher doses can cause nerve damage. If you are pregnant or breastfeeding, or suffer from gout, diabetes, or liver problems, or you have had a stomach ulcer, speak to your GP or pharmacist before taking a vitamin B complex supplement.

Available as: Tablets (e.g. Solgar B-Complex with Vitamin C Stress Formula) and caplets (e.g. Holland & Barrett Complete B Vitamin B Complex caplets).

Check the benefits

To decide whether it is worth continuing to take a supplement, check the effects it is having on your stress levels. Evaluate your stress levels on a scale of nought to ten before supplementation and then repeat after three months of use.

Chapter 7

Relax with DIY Complementary Therapies

The main difference between complementary therapies (also known as alternative, natural or holistic therapies) and conventional Western medicine is that the former focuses on treating the individual as a whole, and identifying and rectifying the causes of illness, whereas the latter concentrates mainly on treating symptoms.

Complementary practitioners believe illness shows that physical and mental well-being have been disrupted, and aim to restore good health by stimulating the body's own self-healing and self-regulating abilities. They claim that total well-being can only be achieved when the mind and body are in a state of balance, called homeostasis. Homeostasis is achieved by following the type of lifestyle advocated in this book, i.e. a healthy diet, with plenty of fresh air, exercise, sleep and relaxation, combined with a positive mental attitude.

Whether complementary therapies work or not remains under debate. Some argue that any benefits are due to the placebo effect. This is where a treatment brings about improvements because the person using it expects it to, rather than because it has any real effect. However, it could be argued that, unlike drug treatments, which are relatively recent, complementary therapies like aromatherapy, massage and reflexology have been used to treat ailments and promote well-being for thousands of years.

This chapter offers a brief overview and evaluation of complementary therapies that can help you to relax and unwind, to help counterbalance the negative effects of stress. You'll find simple techniques and treatments to help you return to calm, including acupressure, aromatherapy, massage, Bach flower remedies, homeopathy, meditation, reflexology and emotional freedom technique (EFT).

What happens in your body when you relax?

 Parasympathetic nervous system takes over.

 Levels of adrenaline and cortisol fall.

 Breathing deepens and slows down.

 Heart rate slows down.

 Muscles loosen.

 Pupils go back to normal.

 Salivation goes back to normal.

 Blood vessels return to normal.

 Blood pressure drops.

 Blood sugar levels drop.

 Cholesterol levels fall.

Production of white blood cells slows down.

 Sweat glands close.

Digestion returns to normal.

 Bladder contracts.

Feeling of calm.

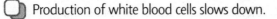

44. Apply acupressure

Like acupuncture, acupressure is part of traditional Chinese medicine and is often described as 'acupuncture without needles', as it stimulates the same points on the body. Both acupressure and acupuncture are based on the idea that life energy, or qi, flows through 22 channels in the body known as meridians. An even passage of qi throughout the body is viewed as essential for good health. Disruption of the flow of qi in a meridian can lead to illness at any point within it. The flow of qi can be affected by various factors, including stress, emotional distress, diet and environment.

Using the fingers and thumbs to apply firm but gentle pressure to points known as acupoints is claimed to remove energy blockages and stimulate the body's natural self-healing abilities. Muscular tension is relieved and circulation boosted, thereby promoting good health. Although it may seem hard to believe something so simple can make a difference, it's important to remember that acupressure has been used for thousands of years and many Chinese people still use it to self-treat a range of common conditions. An animal study in 2011 found that acupuncture reduced levels of the protein neuropeptide Y, which is released during the 'fight or flight' response. Also, there is scientific evidence that stimulating particular acupoints can relieve pain, and several studies back the use of acupuncture for a range of other conditions.

It's thought that the application of pressure stimulates the production of endorphins and encephalins (pain-relieving hormones). You can try the following simple stress-relieving acupressure techniques for yourself:

- **Seal hall** – Also known as yin tang, or the third eye point, this acupoint is found between the eyebrows, in the indentation where the bridge of the nose joins the forehead. Use both index fingers to apply firm pressure to this area for up to two minutes to relieve stress and tension, and induce calm.

- **Shoulder well** – Also known as jian jing, this acupoint is situated on top of each shoulder muscle, half way between the tip of the shoulder and the spine. Apply firm pressure using your index and middle fingers to relieve tension and irritability, and ease muscular pain in the neck and shoulders.

- **Sea of tranquility** – Also known as shanchung, this acupoint is located in the middle of the breastbone, three thumb widths up from the bottom of the bone. To relieve tension, close your eyes, and breathe slowly and deeply as you press on this area with both index fingers, and imagine all of your worries floating away.

45. Find relief in reflexology

Reflexology is based on the theory that points on the feet, hands and face, known as reflexes, correspond to different parts of the body, such as glands and organs, linked via vertical zones along which energy flows. Illness is due to these zones becoming blocked. Stimulating the reflexes using the fingers and thumbs is claimed to bring about physiological changes that remove these blockages, and encourage the mind and body to self-heal.

Practitioners believe that imbalances in the body cause granular deposits in the relevant reflex, which leads to tenderness. Corns, bunions, and even hard skin, are all believed to signify problems in the related parts of the body. The energy theory behind reflexology is very similar to the one underpinning acupressure, although practitioners say it is a different system. There is no scientific evidence that reflexology relieves stress, but there is anecdotal evidence that it is relaxing.

A reflexologist will usually work on your feet because they believe the feet are more sensitive. However, it's usually easier to work on your hands when you are self-treating.

Try the techniques below for instant relaxation and stress relief:

Release tension and refocus your mind
Using your left thumb, gently press down on the solar plexus reflex in the middle of your right palm and rotate anti-clockwise for one minute. Now repeat on your left hand using your right thumb.

Relieve stress and worry
Using your left thumb and index finger, squeeze the top half of your right thumb, where the brain reflex is located. Repeat on your left thumb, using your right thumb and index finger.

Relax and relieve panic

Using your left thumb, apply pressure along the diaphragm line on your right hand. The diaphragm line starts three-quarters of the way up the inside edge of your palm (beneath your little finger) and runs straight across to the outer edge of your palm (beneath your index finger). Repeat on your left hand using your right thumb.

46. Tap away stress

Like acupuncture and acupressure, the emotional freedom techniques (EFT) are energy therapies based on meridian theory – the idea that energy channels run through the body. According to EFT, many of us hold on to negative emotions, which are then stored in the meridians, where they disrupt the flow of energy and cause more negative thoughts. The technique is derived from the Chinese system of chi kung, which involves tapping on particular points to rebalance the energy flow throughout the body.

In EFT you repeat a statement that describes your negative emotions in a way that makes you feel more positive, while tapping particular points on your meridians. It is claimed that this sends a pulse of energy through the meridians, which releases your negative emotions. A similar technique, called thought field therapy, has been adapted and used by the hypnotherapist Paul McKenna to help people overcome stress, anxiety and food cravings. Celebrity fans of the technique include Madonna and Lily Allen. Try these three steps to tap away stress:

1. Describe how you feel, for example: 'I feel really stressed out' or 'I'm stressed to breaking point'. Next, to help you feel more

positive about yourself, reframe this statement with the words 'Even though… I deeply love and approve of myself', so that the statement becomes: 'Even though I feel really stressed out, I deeply love and approve of myself'.

2. Using the tips of your index and middle fingers, tap five times on the 'side of eye' meridian points, situated on the outer bony part of the eye socket where the eyebrows end. Stimulating this point is said to promote calm. As you tap, repeat your statement, so that you focus on the stressed feelings you want to eradicate.

3. Using your right index and middle fingers, tap five times on the left 'underarm' meridian point, situated under your armpit, in line with your nipple. Repeat on your right side using your left index and middle fingers. Stimulating these points is said to relieve worry, aid concentration and speed up thought processes. As you tap, repeat your statement to help you focus on the worry you want to eradicate.

For more information and an EFT tapping points diagram go to www.theenergytherapycentre.co.uk/tapping-points.htm.

47. Use aroma power

Oils with antidepressant, sedative or stimulating properties are particularly helpful during times of stress. Essential oils are extracted using various methods – steam distillation being the commonest – from the petals, leaves, stalk, roots, seeds, nuts and even the bark of plants. Aromatherapy is based on the belief that inhaling the scents released from essential oils affects the hypothalamus, the part of the brain that governs the glands and hormones, thus altering mood, and lowering stress and anxiety. When used in massage, baths and compresses, the oils are also absorbed through the bloodstream and transported to the organs and glands, which benefit from their healing effects.

Massage oil

In massage oil a two per cent dilution is normally used: this equates to two drops per teaspoon of carrier oil. Stronger oils may need more dilution – this is mentioned where necessary below. Sweet almond and grapeseed oils are popular carrier oils. You can also use good-quality olive, sunflower or sesame oil from your kitchen. See below for more about massage.

Never apply aromatherapy oils to broken skin. Buy the best quality essential oils you can afford; like most things, you get what you pay for – cheaper oils may not be as pure as more expensive ones and are more likely to be mixed with solvents or synthetic oils. If you have sensitive skin it is a good idea to do a patch test before using an essential oil you haven't used before. Apply a few drops of diluted oil inside a wrist or an elbow. If there is no reaction within 24 hours it should be safe to go ahead and use the oil.

Soak in a stress-relieving aromatic bath

Fill the bath with comfortably hot water. When you are ready to get in, add six drops of your chosen essential oil (unless otherwise stated). Stir the water around with your hand to spread the oil, which will form a thin film on the water. The warmth of the water both aids absorption through the skin and releases aromatic vapours, which are then inhaled.

Steam inhalation

This method is good for headaches, or for when you feel you need to clear your head. Add three or four drops of your chosen oil to a bowl of very hot, but not boiling, water. Lean over the bowl and carefully drape a large towel around your head and the bowl. Now inhale the vapours for a minute or two.

Caution: Supervise children while using this method, to ensure they don't scald themselves.

Make a compress

A hot compress is a great way of relieving stress-related muscular pain, especially in the neck, shoulders and back, and also works well for headaches. Sprinkle four or five drops of your chosen oil to a basin of hot water and soak a facecloth or men's handkerchief. Wring out the excess moisture and apply to the painful area.

Relaxing and mood-boosting oils

According to Patricia Davis, author of *Aromatherapy – An A–Z*, sedative and antidepressant oils like bergamot, chamomile, lavender, neroli and rose help to both relax you and lift your mood.

 Bergamot – with its citrussy aroma, is uplifting, yet at the same time relaxing and soothing.

(Caution: use in one per cent dilution – in higher strengths it can increase your skin's sensitivity to sunlight and the risk of burning.)

Chamomile (Roman and German) – soothing, calming, relieves irritability, nervousness and insomnia, and boosts mood.

Lavender – balances moods, calms, eases stress, and relieves headaches and insomnia. One of its active ingredients is linalool, which is thought to stimulate brain receptors for GABA, a brain chemical that induces calm. Japanese researchers recently claimed that inhaling lavender oil for five minutes daily dramatically reduces levels of the stress hormone cortisol.

 Neroli (orange blossom) – has a floral, citrusy scent that has a calming effect, making it useful for easing short-term stress, e.g. before an exam or job interview. It also helps long-term stress – especially if it is causing insomnia.

 Rose – balances emotions, eases feelings of grief and loss, and helps with premenstrual syndrome (PMS).

Stimulating oils

According to Davis, stimulating oils such as black pepper, geranium, peppermint and rosemary strengthen the action of the adrenal glands, and help to relieve stress-induced physical and mental exhaustion. Don't use these oils near bedtime as they may cause restlessness and insomnia.

 Black pepper – a general tonic and stimulant, eases muscular pain and helps to relieve irritable bowel syndrome (IBS) when massaged into the tummy area, or applied on a warm compress.

 Geranium – lifts mood and balances hormones.

 Peppermint – assists clear thinking, relieves headaches, including migraines, and tummy upsets, including irritable bowel syndrome, when massaged into stomach area; Davis advises using it well diluted – one drop per teaspoon of carrier oil.

Rosemary – boosts memory and concentration, relieves muscular pain.

48. Massage away stress

Massage involves touch – which can help to reduce stress and tension as well as physical pain. It's thought to work by stimulating the release of serotonin and endorphins. According to a study in 2010 at Cedars-Sinai Medical Centre in Los Angeles, massage also boosts immunity and raises levels of oxytocin, promoting contentment and lowering the level of stress hormones in the blood. Massage is also good for easing the stress-related muscular tension that accumulates in the neck and shoulders; it loosens and stretches the muscles and boosts blood circulation. Ask your partner or a friend to give you a massage and then offer to reciprocate; according to Dr Kerstin Uvnäs Moberg, author of *The Oxytocin Factor: Tapping the Hormone of Calm, Love and Healing*, the person giving the massage also benefits from raised levels of oxytocin. Below are some key massage techniques:

Stroking/effleurage – move both hands over the skin in rhythmic fanning or circular movements.

Kneading – use alternate hands to squeeze then release the flesh.

Friction – use your thumbs to apply even pressure to static points, or make small circles.

Hacking – use the sides of your hands alternately to deliver short, sharp taps all over.

Listening to relaxing music during a massage may help to enhance the feelings of relaxation; a study in 2008, involving 236 pregnant women, claimed that listening to classical music helped to relieve stress, anxiety and depression during pregnancy.

Neck and shoulder self-massage

This is a simple self-massage technique that focuses on your neck and shoulders, where tension tends to accumulate.

1. Lift your shoulders as high as you can, as you inhale through your nose.

2. Hold for a count of five, then roll them back and down, as you exhale.

3. Repeat three times.

4. Using your left hand, squeeze the muscles on the right side of your neck.

5. Repeat on the left side, using your right hand.

6. Press the forefinger and middle finger of each hand into either side of the back of your neck.

7. With small circular movements work your way up to the base of your skull.

49. Use flower power

Flower essences have been used for their healing properties for thousands of years. However, it was Dr Edward Bach, a Harley Street doctor, bacteriologist and homeopath, who developed their use in the twentieth century. Bach believed that negative emotions were the root cause of illness. He identified 38 basic negative states of mind and designed a plant or flower-based remedy for each. The remedies are thought to help combat negative emotions, such as fear, despair and uncertainty, but there's only anecdotal evidence regarding their effectiveness.

The remedies are made by infusing flower heads in spring water in direct sunlight, or by boiling twigs from trees, bushes or plants. The infusion is then mixed with brandy (to act as a preservative) to produce a tincture. The remedies can be taken diluted in water, or you can apply them neat to your lips, temples, wrists or behind the ears. They're widely available in pharmacies in handbag-sized 10 ml and 20 ml phials. Below is a list of Bach remedies that you may find helpful when you are feeling stressed.

 Aspen – for illogical fears.

Bach Rescue Remedy – this combination of rock rose, impatiens, clematis, star of Bethlehem and cherry plum is designed to help you cope during times of acute stress, such as before an exam or job interview, and is said to restore inner calm, control and focus. It is also available as a cream, a spray, chewing gum and pastilles.

Clematis – encourages you to focus on the present.

Impatiens – for irritability and tension.

Vervain – for stress caused by perfectionism and doing too much.

White chestnut – for unwanted thoughts, worries and preoccupations.

For further information on how to select a suitable flower remedy, and an online questionnaire that enables you to select a personalised blend, visit www.bachfloweressences.co.uk.

50. Get help with homeopathy

Homeopathy means 'same suffering' and is based on the belief that 'like cures like' – substances that can cause symptoms in a well person can treat the same symptoms in a person who is ill. For example, coffee contains caffeine – excessive amounts of caffeine can over-stimulate the mind and cause nervousness, so the remedy coffea is often prescribed for these very symptoms (see the list of remedies below).

Symptoms such as inflammation or fever are considered a sign that the body is attempting to heal itself. The theory is homeopathic remedies encourage this self-healing process and work in a similar way to vaccines. The substances used in homeopathic remedies come from plant, animal, mineral, bark and metal sources. These substances are made into a tincture, which is then diluted many times over. Paradoxically, homeopaths claim that the more diluted a remedy is, the higher its potency and the lower its potential side effects. They say this is because of the 'memory of water' i.e. the theory that even though the molecules from a substance are diluted, they leave behind an electromagnetic 'footprint' – like a recording on an audiotape – which has an effect on the body.

These ideas are controversial and many medical professionals are sceptical. Evidence to support homeopathy exists, but critics argue that much of it is inconclusive. For example, research published in 2005 found that 71 per cent of patients receiving individualised homeopathy reported 'positive health changes'. The study took place over six years at the Bristol Homeopathic Hospital and involved 6,500 patients with various chronic conditions including depression, headache and chronic fatigue syndrome. Critics of the study argue there was no comparison group and patients may have given a positive response because it was expected.

There are two main types of remedies – whole person based and symptom based. It's probably best to consult a qualified homeopath who will prescribe a remedy aimed at you as a whole person, including your personality, as well as the symptoms you are experiencing. However, if you prefer, you can buy homeopathic remedies at many high street pharmacies and health shops.

Below is a list of homeopathic remedies, along with the stress-related psychological and physical symptoms for which they're commonly recommended. To self-prescribe, simply choose the remedy with indications that most closely match your symptoms. Follow the dosage instructions on the product.

Aurum metallicum
Made from: Gold
Emotional symptoms: Workaholicism; always striving to do more and feeling as though you haven't accomplished as much as you should; and tendency to overreact to criticism.
Physical symptoms: Headaches, palpitations.

Avena sativa
Made from: Oats

Emotional symptoms: Anxiety, inability to concentrate and nervous exhaustion.
Physical symptoms: Exhaustion and chronic insomnia.

Coffea
Made from: Coffee
Emotional symptoms: Racing mind, nervousness and restlessness.
Physical symptoms: Headaches and insomnia caused by overactive brain.

Ignatia amara
Made from: Seeds from the fruit of St Ignatius tree.
Emotional symptoms: Grief, worry, emotional strain and mental stress, made worse by suppressing emotions.
Physical symptoms: Headaches, insomnia and nervous tics.

Nux vomica
Made from: The poison nut tree, which is native to Southeast Asia.
Emotional symptoms: Driven personality, workaholism and irritability.
Physical symptoms: Headaches and irritable bowel syndrome (IBS); premenstrual syndrome (PMS) in women.

Phosphorus
Made from: Mineral found in inorganic phosphate rocks.
Emotional symptoms: Nervousness, fear, restlessness and sensitivity.
Physical symptoms: Nosebleeds, lethargy, palpitations and feeling cold.

Sepia
Made from: Cuttlefish ink.
Emotional symptoms: Feeling unable to cope, weepy and irritable.

Physical symptoms: Headaches, fatigue, and premenstrual syndrome (PMS) in women.

> ### Not a quick fix
>
> Note: practitioners warn that homeopathy isn't a 'quick fix' – the remedies may take some time to take effect. Homeopathic remedies are generally considered safe and don't have any known side effects, although sometimes a temporary worsening of symptoms, known as 'aggravation', can take place. This is viewed as a good sign, as it suggests the remedy is stimulating the healing process. If this happens, stop taking the remedy and wait for your symptoms to improve. If there is steady improvement, don't restart the remedy. If the improvement stops, start taking the remedy again.

This book has offered you lots of ideas on how you can manage stress, and hopefully you are feeling inspired and ready to make some changes to the way you live your life; the following sections aim to help you do this. There are stress-busting recipes to help you put the dietary advice into practice, as well as details of useful products, including the supplements mentioned in Chapter 6, that you may want to try. There is also a list of books you may find helpful if you want to learn more about some of the topics covered in this book. You'll also find the contact details, including the web addresses, of organisations that you may want to consult for further information and support.

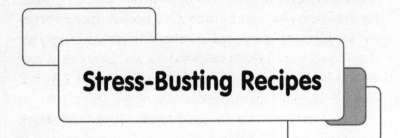

Stress-Busting Recipes

This section contains a selection of recipes based on recommendations for a de-stress diet. They are quick and easy to prepare – perfect for when you're feeling under pressure.

Fruit and seed oat squares (makes around 24 squares)

In this recipe the oats provide slow-release energy and calming tryptophan, while the seeds provide magnesium and zinc, and the wheatgerm supplies selenium. The dried fruits contain calcium and fibre.

Ingredients
170 g rolled oats
55 g wheatgerm
75 g sesame seeds
75 g sunflower seeds
75 g pumpkin seeds
185 g chopped dried fruits (apple, apricot, dates, sultanas)
8 tbsp honey
175 ml boiling water

Method

Line a 3 cm-deep, 16 cm x 28 cm baking tray with baking paper.
Put all of the dry ingredients in a bowl and mix well. Pour the honey
into another bowl. Add the boiling water and stir until the honey has
dissolved. Pour into the oat mixture and mix well. Spoon the mixture
into the lined tray and press down firmly with a spatula. Bake in a
moderate oven until golden brown.

Allow to cool, then cut into small squares. Store in an airtight
container for up to seven days.

Salmon with pepper and onion salsa (serves 1)

In this recipe the salmon provides omega-3 fats and vitamin D
to boost brain function and maintain the immune system during
periods of stress. The pepper, lemon juice, onion and parsley contain
immunity-boosting antioxidants and the chilli has a relaxing effect.

Ingredients

For the salmon
½ tbsp olive oil
150 g salmon fillet, cut into 0.5 cm thick pieces
Juice of half a lemon

For the salsa
¼ yellow pepper
¼ medium red onion
1 tsp chilli flakes
2 tbsp flat leaf parsley
1 tbsp olive oil
Zest and juice of 1 lemon

Method
Salmon

Heat olive oil in a small frying pan on a high heat and fry the salmon slices for 20 seconds on each side, or until just cooked. Put the salmon on a serving plate and squeeze lemon juice over it.

Salsa

Finely chop the pepper, onion and parsley. Mix with the other ingredients in a bowl. Serve with the salmon.

Brown rice risotto (suitable for vegetarians, serves 2)

This recipe contains brown rice, which provides B vitamins and complex carbohydrates to support the nervous system and stabilise the blood sugar. The vegetables also provide complex carbohydrates, amino acids, vitamins and minerals.

Ingredients

1 tbsp olive oil
1 medium onion
½ de-seeded red pepper
200 g brown rice, washed and drained
1 tbsp light soy sauce
1 rounded tsp yeast extract (Marmite)
400 ml water
100 g canned sweetcorn
100 g frozen peas
2 handfuls any mixed fresh herbs, e.g. flat leaf parsley, basil, chervil and coriander
Sea salt and freshly ground black pepper
200 g sunflower seeds

Method

Heat the oil in a large saucepan. Chop the onion and red pepper and fry for 2-3 minutes, until soft. Add the brown rice and cook, stirring continuously, for 1-2 minutes. Put the soy sauce and Marmite into a saucepan on a medium heat and add the hot water, stirring briskly to dissolve. Add to the rice and bring to the boil. Reduce the heat to simmer for about 15 minutes. Add the sweetcorn and peas, and simmer for a further 20-25 minutes, or until the rice is tender.

Finely chop the fresh herbs and stir in. Season with freshly ground black pepper.

Smoked mackerel pate with orange and watercress salad (serves 4)

In this recipe the mackerel provides mood-boosting omega-3 fats and vitamin D. The low-fat cream cheese and natural yogurt contain calming calcium. Watercress is rich in antioxidants, beta-carotene, vitamins B1, B6, C and E, as well as iron, magnesium and zinc.

Ingredients

For the mackerel
6 mackerel fillets, skins removed
150 g low-fat cream cheese
50 g natural set yogurt
Juice and zest of 1 large lemon
A pinch of ground black pepper
A small pinch of cayenne pepper
2 tbsp chopped fresh flat leaf parsley

For the watercress salad
2 bunches of watercress
3 oranges
250 g walnuts
2 tbsp of extra-virgin olive oil

Method
Mash the mackerel fillets with a fork, then mix with low-fat cream cheese and natural set yogurt in a bowl. Add the lemon zest and juice, black pepper, cayenne pepper and parsley, and mix together. Wash the watercress and remove any large stalks. Place in a bowl and set aside. Cut the top and bottom off each orange and stand upright on a chopping board. Remove the peel and pith with a sharp knife, then cut into segments. Gently toss the orange segments with the watercress. Add the extra-virgin olive oil, walnuts and a pinch of ground black pepper. Serve with wholemeal toast.

Pan-fried lamb's liver with carrot salad (serves 1)

Liver is an extremely nutritious food that is often overlooked. In this recipe it provides protein, vitamins A, C and D, and vitamin B complex, as well as zinc, iron and selenium, for healthy nervous and immune systems. The carrots and orange provide the antioxidants beta-carotene and vitamin C, as well as soluble fibre. The olive oil provides monounsaturated fats and is anti-inflammatory.

Ingredients

For the liver
100 g lamb's liver
1 tbsp olive oil
Sea salt and freshly ground black pepper

For the carrot salad
2 large carrots, peeled
3 tbsp olive oil
½ orange, zest and juice
2 tbsp chopped fresh chives

Method
Slice the lamb's liver into 2.5 cm strips, removing any gristle. Heat the olive oil and fry the lamb's liver until browned on the outside and lightly cooked on the inside. Season with a little sea salt and some freshly ground black pepper. Grate the carrots. Beat the olive oil, orange zest, juice and chopped chives together in a bowl, then pour over the carrots and mix in lightly.

Place the carrot salad on a plate, top with the lamb's liver and serve.

Thai green chicken and butternut squash curry (serves 4)

In this recipe the chicken and brown rice provide slow-release energy, protein, fibre, B vitamins and calming tryptophan. The butternut squash and green beans provide immunity-boosting antioxidant vitamins, while the red chilli aids relaxation.

Ingredients
500 g chicken
1 tbsp olive oil
500 g butternut squash, peeled and cut into 1½ cm cubes
100 g trimmed green (French) beans, cut in half
1 clove garlic, finely chopped
2 tbsp Thai green curry paste

2 tbsp Thai fish sauce
400 ml can of light coconut milk
1 large red chilli, deseeded and finely chopped
Fresh coriander
300 g brown rice
1 tbsp olive oil

Method

Place the brown rice in a saucepan of boiling water and cook as per instructions on pack. Heat the olive oil in a large non-stick frying pan or wok, add the chicken and stir-fry for about 4 minutes. Add the butternut squash, green (French) beans and garlic, and stir-fry for a further 3 minutes. Add the chopped chilli, Thai green curry paste, fish sauce, light coconut milk and 100 ml water. Bring to the boil, cover and simmer for about 15 minutes. Sprinkle with the fresh coriander and serve with the cooked brown rice.

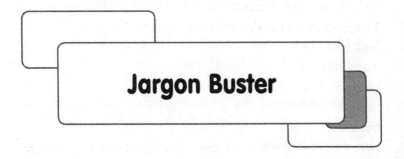

Jargon Buster

Below are explanations of medical terms you'll encounter many times throughout this book:

 Adrenaline – a hormone released by adrenal glands during the stress response.

Antioxidants – substances thought to neutralise free radicals.

 Autoimmune disease – any condition where the body produces antibodies that attack normal tissue.

Cortisol – a hormone released by the adrenal glands during the stress response.

Dopamine – a neurotransmitter involved in feelings of pleasure.

 Endorphins – the body's own painkillers.

Free radicals – substances produced by normal chemical reactions in the body and linked to cell damage.

Gamma-aminobutyric acid (GABA) – a neurotransmitter or brain chemical that promotes calm by reducing brain activity.

 Glycaemic index – a ranking of foods according to the effect they have on blood sugar levels.

Inflammation – the immune system's natural response to irritation, infection or injury. Symptoms include redness, heat, swelling and pain.

Insulin – hormone secreted by the pancreas that lowers blood sugar by directing it into the body's cells.

Melatonin – the 'body clock' hormone that regulates sleep and waking.

Oxytocin – a hormone that promotes contentment and lowers the level of stress hormones in the blood.

Serotonin – a neurotransmitter involved in mood, relaxation, appetite and sleep.

Tryptophan – an amino acid the body uses to make serotonin.

Terms used when referring to clinical trials:

Double-blind – a trial where information that might influence the behaviour of the investigators, or the participants, is withheld, e.g. which participants have been given a placebo, rather than an active substance.

Placebo – an inactive substance given to study participants to compare its effects against those of a treatment.

 Placebo effect – a situation where a person taking a placebo feels better because they believe they have received a treatment and expect to feel better.

Randomised controlled trials (RCTs) – viewed as the most reliable type of research trial because they randomly place participants in a treatment group, or a control group. The treatment group receives the treatment under scrutiny, while the control group receives a placebo or another treatment, for comparison. RCTs can be single blind, where the participant doesn't know which treatment they are receiving, or double-blind, where neither the participants nor the researchers know who is receiving which treatment.

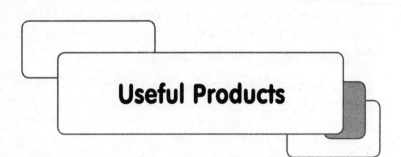

Useful Products

Below is a list of products and suppliers of products that may help to ease stress. The author doesn't endorse or recommend any particular product and this list is by no means exhaustive.

Bach Rescue Remedy
A combination of five Bach Original Flower Remedies blended to help people face daily stresses or emergency situations in a better frame of mind.
Website: www.bachcentre.com

Colour breathing book kit and audio CD
A 'self-relaxation' kit based on colour therapy and breathing that includes a full-colour book with a set of the seven colour breathing discs and an audio CD.
Website: www.colourbreathing.com

Dormeasan Valerian-Hops Oral Drops 50 ml
Registered herbal tincture containing valerian and hops, thought to relieve stress, calm and relax. Also provides relief from stress-related sleep disturbances.
Website: www.avogel.co.uk

G Baldwin & Co
Herbalist founded in London in 1844. Offers a wide range of herbal supplements, tinctures and teabags.
Website: www.baldwins.co.uk

Good 'N Natural Ashwagandha Extract Tablets
Tablets containing 300 mg of ashwagandha extract.
Website: www.hollandandbarrett.com

Herbs for Healing
A Gloucester-based company with an online shop selling medicinal plants and dried herbs, as well as herbal bath and skin products, and the equipment and ingredients to make your own. The website also offers useful information about the medicinal properties of herbs and herbal recipes.
Website: www.herbsforhealing.net

Health Aid Siberian Ginseng Liquid 50 ml
Herbal liquid derived from organically grown herbs. Taken in a small amount of warm water.
Website: www.healthaid.co.uk

Holland & Barrett L-lysine 1,000 mg
Caplets supplying 1,000 mg of L-lysine in a form that is easy for the body to absorb.
Website: www.hollandandbarrett.com

Holland & Barrett L-tyrosine Capsules 500 mg
Capsules containing 500 mg of L-tryosine.
Website: www.hollandandbarrett.com

Kalms
A herbal remedy for anxiety, irritability and stress, containing valerian, gentian and hops.
Website: www.kalmsstress.com

Lamberts Healthcare Ltd
A leading supplier of specialist high-quality dietary supplements.
Website: www.lamberts.co.uk

Lifeplan Siberian Ginseng
Tablets containing 600 mg of Siberian ginseng. Free from added sugar, salt, starch, lactose, gluten, live yeasts, synthetic flavours, artificial colours or preservatives. Suitable for vegans.
Website: www.lifeplan.co.uk

L-tyrosine 500 mg by Biovea
Improves mental alertness, increases feelings of well-being and offsets physical and mental fatigue.
Website: www.biovea.co.uk

Napiers Skullcap, Oat & Passionflower Compound
A classic nerve tonic, containing a range of calming herbs, including skullcap, oats and passion flower, and valerian.
Website: www.napiers.net

Nature's Answer Rhodiola Root Alcohol Free Extract 30 ml
An alcohol-free fluid extract of Rhodiola root.
Website: www.baldwins.co.uk

Nature's Best Pure L-lysine – 500 mg
Tablets providing 500 mg of L-lysine in an easily absorbed form.
Website: www.naturesbest.co.uk

Nelson's Homeopathic Pharmacy
Online shop selling homeopathic remedies, including a combination for nervous anxiety that includes arsenicum album, aconite and gelsemium. Also sells Bach Original Flower Remedies.
Website: www.nelsonshomeopathy.com

Passiflora and Valerian Plus 50 ml

Alcohol-free liquid extract to aid relaxation and sleep. Contains passiflora (passion flower), valerian, Californian poppy, hawthorn and linden.
Website: www.esinaturalhealth.co.uk

Pukka Organic Ashwagandha

Capsules containing organic ashwagandha.
www.pukkaherbs.com

Quiet Life

Tablets containing B vitamins, valerian, hops, passiflora, wild lettuce and motherwort.
Website: www.laneshealth.com

RelaxHerb Passion Flower Extract 425 mg

Supplement containing pharmaceutical-grade extract of passion flower to relieve symptoms of stress, such as mild anxiety.
Website: www.schwabepharma.co.uk

Sibergin 2,500 mg

Capsules containing 2,500 mg of concentrated Siberian ginseng root extract.
Website: www.healthaid.co.uk

Solgar B-Complex with Vitamin C Stress Formula

Gluten-, wheat- and dairy-free tablets containing B complex vitamins and vitamin C.
Website: www.solgar.co.uk

Solgar L-arginine 500 mg Vegetable Capsules

Vegetable capsules free from corn, yeast, soy, wheat, gluten and dairy.
Website: www.solgar.co.uk

Solgar Siberian Ginseng Root Extract

Contains powdered Siberian ginseng root and powder, and standardised root extract.
Website: www.solgar.co.uk

The Stress Dot Card

A credit card-sized card with dots that monitor your stress levels by changing colour according to the temperature of your hands and feet, which reflects how stressed you are.
Website: www.stresscheck.co.uk

Stressless

Tablets harnessing the sedative properties of hops, skullcap, valerian and vervain, to help relieve stress.
Website: www.hollandandbarrett.com

Tisserand Aromatherapy

This company offers a wide range of good quality essential oils designed to improve health and happiness.
Telephone: 01273 325666
Email: sales@tisserand.com
Website: www.tisserand.com

Viridian Maximum Potency Rhodiola Rosea Root Extract Vegicaps

Vegetarian capsules containing 250 mg of standardised rhodiola rosea root extract. Free from gluten, wheat, lactose, added sugar, salt, yeast, preservatives or artificial colourings.

Vitano

A supplement containing pharmaceutical-grade standardised extract of rhodiola rosea to relieve mild anxiety, stress and exhaustion.
Website: www.schwabepharma.co.uk

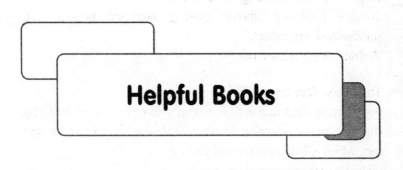

Helpful Books

Alexander, Jane, *The Overload Solution: How to Stop Juggling and Start Living* (Piatkus, 2005) – this book explains how overload affects our health and relationships, and suggests ways to beat it and reclaim your life.

Austin, Denise, *Pilates For Every Body: Strengthen, Lengthen and Tone Your Body* (Rodale, 2002) – a useful guide to Pilates with various routines lasting five or ten minutes, including one for beginners.

Davis, Patricia, *Aromatherapy: An A–Z* (Vermillion, 2005) – a comprehensive guide to essential oils and how to use them to relieve stress and improve your well-being.

James, Dr Oliver, *Affluenza* (Vermilion, 2007) – this book offers an interesting perspective on the increase in what the author calls 'emotional distress', arguing that excessive materialism is to blame, and that the antidote is to be grateful for what you have and buying what you need, rather than what you want.

Tolle, Eckhart, *The Power of Now* (Hodder & Stoughton, 1999) – a thought-provoking guide to dealing with the pressures of twenty-first-century living, by staying focused on the present rather than worrying about the past or the future.

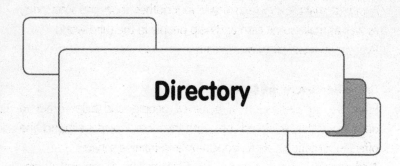

Directory

Below is a list of contacts offering useful information and support when you are suffering from stress.

ABC of Yoga
A website offering tips, advice and poses for those who wish to practise yoga at home. Also provides meditation techniques.
Website: www.abc-of-yoga.com

The Body Control Pilates Association
A website where you can learn about Pilates, find a Pilates teacher and buy equipment.
Website: www.bodycontrol.co.uk

Citizens Advice Bureau
Helps people resolve their legal, financial, emotional and other problems by providing free, independent and confidential advice. Visit the website for online advice and contact details for your local CAB.
Registered office: Myddelton House, 115–123 Pentonville Road, London N1 9LZ
Website: www.citizensadvice.org.uk

Clothes for Cash

A website that allows you to recycle your clothes, shoes and accessories, as well as make some cash and help people in the third world.

Website: www.clothesforcash.com

Cruse Bereavement Care

Promotes the well-being of bereaved people, and helps them to understand their grief and cope with their loss. Provides support and offers information, advice, education and training services.

Address: Cruse Bereavement Care, PO Box 800, Richmond, Surrey TW9 2RG

Telephone: 0844 477 9400

Email: helpline@cruse.org.uk

Website: www.crusebereavementcare.org.uk

Freecycle

An online recycling organisation that aims to reduce waste, save resources and ease the burden on landfill sites by encouraging people to give and get unwanted items for free.

Website: www.freecycle.org

Freegle

A recycling organisation that aims to keep anything reusable out of landfill sites by encouraging people to give away and receive unwanted items for free.

Website: www.ilovefreegle.org

Health Supplements Information Service

Service that aims to provide accurate and balanced information on vitamins, minerals and food supplements.

Address: 52a Cromwell Road, London SW7 5BE

Email: info@hsis.org

Website: www.hsis.org

International Stress Management UK
ISMA[UK] is a registered charity and the leading professional body representing a multi-disciplinary professional health and well-being membership in the UK and the ROI. It promotes sound knowledge and best practice in the prevention and reduction of human stress. It also sets professional standards for the benefit of individuals and organisations using the services of its members.
Telephone: 0845 680 7083
Email: stress@isma.org.uk
Website: www.isma.org.uk

Medicines and Healthcare Products Regulatory Agency (MHRA)
A government agency responsible for ensuring that medicines and medical devices work, and are acceptably safe.
Address: 151 Buckingham Palace Road, Victoria, London SW1W 9SZ
Telephone: 020 3080 6000
Email: info@mhra.gsi.gov.uk
Website: www.mhra.gov.uk

Mental Health Foundation
UK charity that provides helpful information and carries out research on the causes, prevention and treatment of mental health problems, including stress and stress-related disorders. The foundation also campaigns for, and works to improve, services for anyone affected by mental health problems. It takes an integrated approach to mental health that incorporates both social and biological factors. Online resources include downloadable podcasts on stress and relaxation. The charity's Be Mindful campaign offers information on reducing your stress levels using mindfulness, an online mindfulness course and details of mindfulness courses across the UK.
Address: Mental Health Foundation, London Office, 9th Floor, Sea Containers House, 20 Upper Ground, London SE1 9QB
Telephone: 020 7803 1100

Email: mhf@mhf.org.uk

Websites: www.mentalhealth.org.uk, www.bemindful.co.uk

Mind

A national charity for emotional and mental health problems – including those resulting from stress; offers information and advice online and through a network of local Mind associations that offer counselling, befriending, drop-in sessions etc.

Address: 15-19 Broadway, Stratford, London E15 4BQ

Telephone: 020 8519 2122

Mind Information Line: 08457 660163 (local rate, Monday to Friday, 9.15 a.m.–5.15 p.m.)

Email: contact@mind.org.uk

Website: www.mind.org.uk

The Money Advice Service

An organisation that provides advice on a range of financial issues, including managing your money, dealing with debt, savings, mortgages and pensions; the website contains a host of tools and advice to help you take control of your finances.

Telephone: Money Advice Line – 0300 500 5000, Monday to Friday, 8 a.m.–6 p.m. (except bank holidays); typetalk 18001 0300 500 5000

Address: The Money Advice Service, 25 The North Colonnade, Canary Wharf, London E14 5HS

Email: enquiries@moneyadviceservice.org.uk

Website: www.moneyadviceservice.org.uk

Money Saving Expert

A website dedicated to saving people money on anything and everything, by finding the best deals and beating the system. Created and owned by leading financial journalist Martin Lewis.

Website: www.moneysavingexpert.com

National Debtline

Offers free confidential and independent advice on how to deal with debt problems.

Address: Tricorn House, 51–53 Hagley Road, Edgbaston, Birmingham B16 8TP

Telephone: 0808 808 4000

Website: www.nationaldebtline.co.uk

NHS Direct

NHS website offering an online Initial Assessment, where you can check your symptoms and get health advice. The website also links to NHS Choices, which has a 'healthy living' section with advice on dealing with stress, including specialist advice on dealing with stress caused by the credit crunch. You can also find out about psychological therapy services, such as counselling and CBT, near you. Useful online tools include workplace stress and 'mental health' and 'lift your mood' video walls, where people share their experiences via video clips. There are also blogs and forums on specific health topics (NHS Choices Talk), including mental health issues, such as stress and anxiety.

NHS Stressline: 0300 123 2000 (8 a.m.–10 p.m., seven days a week)

Website: www.nhsdirect.nhs.uk

Really Worried

A website where you can you can seek or share help and advice on just about any worrying topic.

Website: www.reallyworried.com

Relate

With 2,500 professionally trained counsellors, Relate is the UK's largest provider of relationship counselling and sex therapy. The charity offers counselling, sex therapy and relationship education to support couple and family relationships throughout life. Visit the

website for helpful relationship advice, to find your nearest Relate, or to consult a counsellor by email. Alternatively, you can arrange counselling by telephone.
Telephone: 0300 100 1234
Website: www.relate.org.uk

Relaxation for Living Institute

A charity that offers information on stress and its effects on the body, as well as relaxation techniques. Also provides a database of Relaxation for Living Institute teachers and relaxation classes across the UK.
Address: Relaxation for Living Institute, 1 Great Chapel Street, London W1F 8FA
Telephone: 020 7439 4277
Website: www.rfli.co.uk

Samaritans

A UK charity that offers confidential non-judgemental emotional support, 24 hours a day, to people experiencing feelings of distress or despair, including those that could lead to suicide. This service is available over the telephone, by email, face to face or by letter.
Address: Chris, PO Box 9090, Stirling FK8 2SA
Telephone: 08457 909090
Email: jo@samaritans.org
Website: www.samaritans.org

The Stress Management Society

The Stress Management Society is a non-profit-making organisation dedicated to helping people tackle stress. The website offers a wealth of information about stress and how to deal with it.
Telephone: 0844 357 8629
Email: info@stress.org.uk
Website: www.stress.org.uk

Have you enjoyed this book?
If so, why not write a review on your favourite website?

Thanks very much for buying this Summersdale book.

www.summersdale.com

@summersdale